Doctor Bison's Fables

An Allegory of the American Pain Refugee Crisis

For permission requests, write to the publisher, addressed
"Attention: Permissions Coordinator"
carol@markvictorhansenlibrary.com

Quantity sales special discounts are available on quantity purchases by corporations, associations, and others. For details, contact the publisher at
carol@markvictorhansenlibrary.com

Orders by U.S. trade bookstores and wholesalers.
Email: carol@markvictorhansenlibrary.com

Creative contribution by J. Collin Phillips
Cover Design - J. Collin Phillips
Illustrations - Matt Phillips
Book Layout - DBree, StoneBear Design

Manufactured and printed in the United States of America distributed globally by
markvictorhansenlibrary.com

MVHL

New York | Los Angeles | London | Sydney

ISBN: 979-8-88581-132-3 Hardback
ISBN: 979-8-88581-133-0 Paperback
ISBN: 979-8-88581-134-7 eBook
Library of Congress Control Number: 9798885811323

DEDICATION

To my children Grace and Alfred:
The lights of my life

And thank you to Susan Franzheim for vision, perspective, coaching and editing.

To the team at Mark Victor Hansen Library for the visionary idea to write a fable. I'm convinced now!

TABLE OF CONTENTS

Pain Refugees 2
Wheelhouse 3
Cast of Characters 4
Prologue 6
Chapter 1 What is a Doctor 11
Chapter 2 The Crowded Room 21
Chapter 3 Relating Too Well 29
Chapter 4 Fear and Superstition 39
Chapter 5 Held Hostage 47
Chapter 6 Breeding Resentment 57
Chapter 7 Higher Calling 69
Chapter 8 The Definition of Pain 77
Chapter 9 Alternative Lifestyles 87
Chapter 10 Pursuing Happiness 97
Chapter 11 Secret Calling 107
Chapter 12 Medical Refugees 119
Chapter 13 The Hole and the Way Out 129
Chapter 14 Do No Harm 139
Epilogue 151
About the Author 152

Pain Refugees

"I am not comfortable providing that treatment."

"Well, it's not for your comfort, it's for the patient's comfort."

Pain casts a shadow.

That darkness, unlike pain, is intangible. But it bleeds, festers.

It gives birth to fear. Unrest. Discomfort. Agony.
The treatment of pain breeds more pain, tainted
by that invisible wrongness.

So, the culture becomes infected by a plague of neglect toward health and healing. Vilifying the very people who only want to heal the pain, reviling the victims of the remedies they become dependent on for succor.

"My hands are tied." The motto of the system: a billing system disguised as medical records, holding health hostage. Mortgages taken out against human lives.

The principal of that loan is wellness.

The interest on that loan is terror.

The cost of defaulting is death.

Wheelhouse

By Mark Ibsen, MD

I stand in the wheelhouse of our humanity,
Responding to reports of calm seas
While navigating a class 4 storm,
And I know that my shipmates and I are
On
Our
Own
And that we will weather this storm, return to port
And
Have something to say to the shore bound
"navigators" who kept lying
To us
About what was right
before our eyes.

Cast of Characters

TOWN LEADERS
Mayor Weasel
Mason Moose, Dr. Bison's benefactor and richest animal in the territory

MEDICAL PERSONNEL
Dr. Bryan Bison
Otis Owl, apothecary
Nurse Rebecca Rabbit
Miss Milly Mole, the town's midwife (Mother Mole)
Mister Ferrett, assigned to doctor's office to make sure patients pay
Miss Vole, Mr. Ferret's secretary
Professor Ermine, Dr. Bison's teacher
Doctor Crane, got his patients hooked on pain meds then left them to suffer when meds ran out
Muskrat, dealing in bad pain meds

PATIENTS
Philip Otter, Senior, local family
Philip Otter Jr., patient
Gill the Billy Goat, patient
Myron Mouse, patient
Mrs. Goat, cranky patient
Emmett Crow, cranky patient
Jack Hare, long eared patient
Finn Fox, patient
Ogle Opossum, patient, cannabis farmer
Mister Goose, elder patient

THE LAW
Judge Falcon
Counselor Coyote, for the prosecution
Counselor Woodchuck, for the defense
Alan Aardvark, former constable and old acquaintance

WESTERN TEAM
Lham Llama, wise llama in the mountains
Silas Sidewinder, friendly rattlesnake
Dr. Louis 'Lou' Labrador, the medical dog
Nurse Squirrel
Cora Cow, herbalist
Moss Stoneherd Elk, warrior in training
Neinoo Stoneherd Elk, tribe leader, medicine cow
Buck, patient in pain
Deadre Deer, wife of Buck

PROLOGUE

This book was generated out of the catastrophic events for my patients and me over the last 10+ years.

The Montana board of medicine from 2013 to 2015 conspired with National officials and perpetrated fraudulent findings.

The cost of this was a pyrrhic victory for me. The IRS seized my assets, the Dream Clinic Urgent Care Plus was shut down. These actions cost me $350,000 in legal fees, and my business and my building. These actions cast a pall over prescribing practices in Montana.

I tried to continue treating pain patients until Dr. Chris Christiansen, 78, was convicted of manslaughter in late 2017. It became clear to me that I was now practicing in a hostile regulatory environment, as the board of medicine reported me to the drug enforcement administration (DEA) and they came to my office to investigate me.

The agent said: "Dr. Ibsen, you're risking your freedom as well as your license by prescribing to Patients like these."

I said, "Patients like whom?"

They said, "Patients who might divert their pain medication."

I said, "Isn't that everyone?" (who might divert or sell their pain meds).

A 1989 cross-roads moment between my white coat and saffron robes, a kind of "Eat, Pray, Love" opportunity in India at an ashram, the leader, Gurumayi, guided me in a private audience:

"What if a baby would fall from the sky?" after noting my baby-faced appearance. And eight years later, my daughter was born.

Next traveling to Kolkata, where as a volunteer for Mother Teresa who described herself as "I am just a pencil in the hand of God."

I incorporated this into my spiritual and medical mission, and newly emerging spiritual life. My comeuppance showed up like this: hotshot ER doc finds himself on the lowest rung of the hierarchy in an international location.

With Mother Teresa in Kolkata, I experienced the oppressive, grinding nature of poverty. I was blowing black stuff out of my nose every evening and black stuff out of my heart every day.

In the Ramayana, the epic spiritual Scripture of Hinduism, Lord Krishna declares to the warrior Arjuna, "Do your duty *and* surrender the fruits of your labor."

In India, I had the opportunity to observe that Saints are not necessarily always surrounded by saintly people.

I was continuously confronted when given an assignment by someone. "Did this come from the guru or Mother Teresa, or did this come from your ego?" Ultimately, I decided it didn't matter, and that I needed to love them all; let God sort them out.

Prior to India, the medical industrial complex controlled my agenda. It was all I knew. In India, I surrendered to Spirit. In the conventional medical model, I had attained a certain confidence.

Did I need to reinvent myself? To show myself that I could? To find a place in which I would?

In response to my query, DEA agent Addis said, "We are not doctors, we can't tell you what to do."

Yet, the charge of over-prescribing is evidence of their de facto practice of medicine, by imposing regulations without guidelines, citations, or evidence. And if I was guilty of over-prescribing, then so were all the doctors who prescribed for these patients before they sought my help.

I was more successful, according to David Scrimm, the administrative law judge supervising the hearings, than the government's expert witness at weaning patients off of opiates. My success rate was 80%. I truly anticipated an award for this accomplishment.

I was exonerated after these hearings, proving that no patient was harmed, most were helped. Parenthetically, one bitter pill from this is that six of my patients died after losing access to my care, not before.

Despite the burden of proof put on me, I was able to demonstrate the treating of pain refugees was not illegal, in fact, it was crucial—a noble calling.

The courtroom loss and my vindication was a bitter pill for the board of medicine to swallow. To save face, their next mission creep was to sanction me for my documentation. Not only were the documents I gave them ultimately out of order, when I reviewed their notes, they criticized my handwriting as illegible. I responded only that "they're encrypted."

I was selected as the best doctor in Helena in 2014, and out of business by 2015.

What's wrong with this picture?

Judge James Reynolds ruling in the District Court appeal, overruled the suspension of my license and found that the board of medicine violated my due process rights.

In 2016, I returned to India as a volunteer with Hands on Global, a local Helena non-governmental organization, (NGO), who were tasked with opening the hospital the Dalai Lama built in Zanskar. This is the last intact Tibetan civilization on the planet and while his Holiness wants the population to make progress in health, he also wants to preserve this precious ancient culture.

When the Dalai Lama came to inspect and celebrate the completion of the hospital, he came into the examining room.

He noticed the ultrasound machine I was using. He said, "Oh, ultrasound, I know this!"

I called his attention to two stuffed pillows I had brought with me; one a yellow Labrador Retriever, and one a kitty cat.

I said, "Your Holiness, we also have labs and CAT scans available!"

He responded, "Ho, ho, ho," as robust as Santa Claus.

Love them all; let God sort them out, continues to inspire me. I have realized that self-pity and resentment are not my friends. As my recovery work progresses, I use more friendly slogans like *let go and let God*.

As a dog musher from 2001 forward, I also learned to let go and let dog!

After Dr. Christianson's conviction on manslaughter charges, I saw the writing on the wall. Montana has become a hostile regulatory environment for me.

I retired from prescribing opiates.

Sadly, six of my patients died after losing access to my care.

I welcome you to *Doctor Bison's Fables*.

CHAPTER ONE

WHAT IS A DOCTOR?

THE BISON AND THE MOUSE

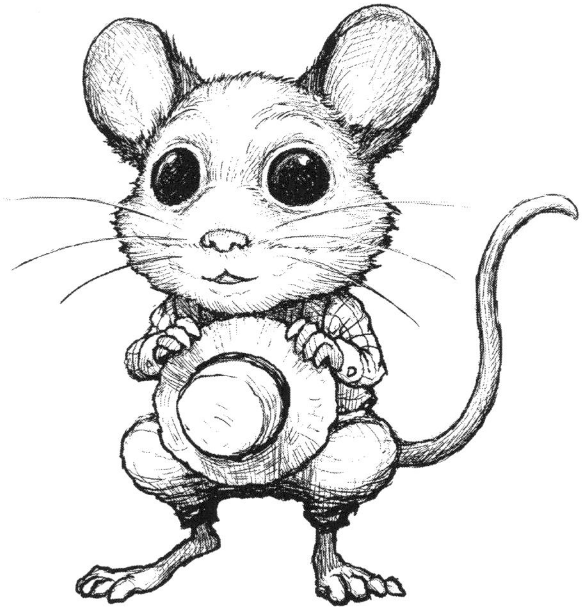

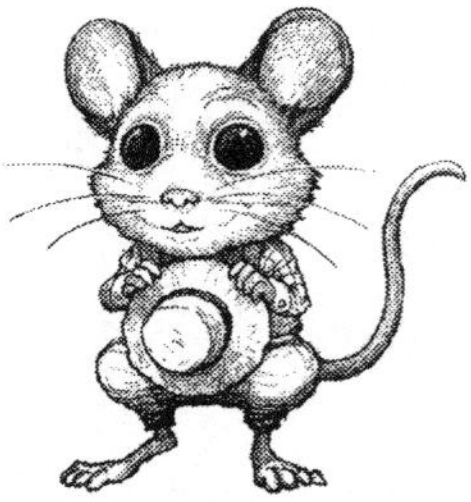

Once upon a time, there lived a bison who wanted to help other animals, and so spent his life studying medicine to become a doctor. So it was that the bison came upon a family of mice who were all sick, but they had nothing with which to pay for the doctor's aid. "But without my care, your children will die. I must help, it is my duty," he said.

Without a thought, the doctor gave them his aid, one after the other, and each mouse he healed was grateful. Soon, however, he began to tire and eventually became exhausted, yet still more mice came. "Surely, though, this deed will be worth it in the end," he thought, and strengthened his resolve.

By morning the bison was falling asleep on his feet, and told the mice, "I am sorry, but I must go rest."

"But sir, we still have more sick children."

The bison saw the line of mice reaching as far as he could see, and he despaired.

Despite their duty, the healer must heal in order to heal others.

"HOW BAD IS IT, DOC?"

"We'll probably have to amputate, Philip." Doctor Bryan Bison turned, an exaggerated, somber scowl on his wide bison face.

The tiny otter's eyes bulged out as he gasped, clutching his worn-out ball to his chest. He shot a glance at his mother, who huffed a little laugh and rested a reassuring hand on his shoulder.

"Yep, that's what they always said when we were growing up. Only cure for a thorn in the paw is to remove the whole foot." Papa Otter sat with his arms crossed in the corner. "It's a wonder we have any limbs left at all."

The big doctor couldn't hide his grin as he sat on the rolling stool and scooted closer to the bench. "Now, can I take a look? I promise I won't start chopping just yet."

Philip grimaced to hide his smile, realizing that he was the butt of the joke. He hissed softly as the doctor gently reached for his foot. "It hurts so bad."

"I know. Once, I had a burr wedged in my hoof for a week. I could barely sleep, it hurt so bad. But you know what? Ignoring it only made it worse. Eventually, it was much more difficult to get out because I just hoped it would go away."

Philip hesitated, shakily extending his leg. No sooner had he stretched it out than he jerked back, seeing the tweezers gleam. "No no no, I'm too scared."

"It's okay, honey. Doctor B knows what he is doing. It will be over so fast." Momma Otter tried to console him.

Across the room, Papa Otter sighed, losing his patience. "Look, if we have to, we'll just hold him down and—"

"Ahem." The doctor cleared his throat a little too loudly, staring pointedly at Papa Otter. The gruff, but much smaller animal sat back down. "No need for all that. I think . . . hmm . . . there may be another way. Completely pain free."

Philips perked up, nodding emphatically.

"I probably shouldn't tell you about this new, experimental procedure."

"Tell me, please, tell me."

"Well, we could just replace your paw with a brand new one."

"Wow, you can do that?"

"Yep. Only thing I need though, is for you to pay for it," he lowered his head to look Philip in the eye. To the side, Momma Otter gave the doctor a sly look.

"Oh, okay. How much does it cost?"

"One old ball."

A look of horror stole over the child's face. He pondered a moment, glancing from his ball to his foot and back. After a moment, resolution slumped his little shoulders as he thrust out his hands holding the ratty leather ball.

Very carefully, and with the utmost reverence, Dr. Bison reached out and took the ball, making a show of placing it into his desk and writing down a receipt on his file chart. Rolling back over he motioned for Philip to extend his foot. The little creature complied and relaxed his paw.

The thorn jutting from the pad of his foot was quite large. But the real concern was the swelling. *Infected*, thought Bryan. *They shouldn't have let it go this long*.

"Alright, look out the window for me for a moment, while I get the new foot ready."

The child complied, holding his mother's paw.

Swiftly, Dr. Bison drew out something from his pocket, setting it in Philip's lap as he applied a swab of iodine simultaneously. The flash of movement brought the little boy's attention back to a new, shiny red ball.

"See? Brand new," the doctor muttered and plucked the thorn

out in a deft motion, immediately pressing a cotton swab to the opening to staunch the blood. Philip only flinched slightly; the ball held aloft in front of his face.

“Whoa! Thank you, Doc B.” The lithe critter rolled forward, throwing one little arm around the bison’s huge neck.

“You’re welcome. Now sit tight, while Nurse Rebecca cleans and wraps it up for you. I need to talk to your mommy and daddy to get you a *potion* to make sure it heals up right.” He rose and guided the otter couple toward his office door as a smiling rabbit in a crisp white nurse outfit entered. Giggles followed them into the office from the examination room.

“Please, sit down. I will prescribe an antibiotic for the infection. You brought him in just in time.”

“How much’ll that cost us, Doc?” Poppa Otter looked down, embarrassed to ask. Everyone in town knew the Otters didn’t have much money.

“Don’t fret about that just yet. Most important thing is to make sure Philip’s paw heals. The infection is pretty far along, but if you keep it clean and he takes his medicine, it should be fine. I’ll want to see him again in a couple of days to make sure it’s closing.”

“Thank you so much Doctor,” Poppa Otter muttered, holding his wife’s hand as she held back tears. “I promise, we will get the money for the bill soon as we get paid for this week’s clam haul.”

“Please, take these. I baked them fresh this morning.” Momma set a basket covered in a worn, but clean cloth on the desk. She wobbled slightly as she sat back, an old injury the doctor knew she had never gotten proper treatment for.

“I will certainly take one of those delicious muffins, Mrs. Otter, but not the whole lot, got to watch my weight, you know.” The big doctor rose, purposefully taking only one of the treats and gently scooting the basket back toward her. "Rebecca will get you settled out front and I will have the medicine ready for you shortly."

The couple smiled graciously, thanking him as they excused themselves.

In the quiet, Bryan sat down, sighing softly. He scribbled absently on a script sheet, unintelligible as always. Nurse Rebecca and the town's chemist and pharmacist, Oliver Owl, always managed to decipher it.

If only I could decipher how to help the Otters pay for this, for medicine, for continued care.

But they weren't the only ones. Half of the town was in no better situation financially.

"Doctor?"

Bryan shook himself, looking up. Rebecca was peering around the door, smirking like she did when she had to call him several times to get his attention.

"Sorry, lost in thought."

"Is that the Otter's script? I'll run over and see that Mister Owl has it ready for them for purchase when they arrive."

"Good, good. Ah, go ahead and tell him to fill the script and we'll work the payment out later."

"Doctor," she chided softly, "Mister Mason won't take kindly to you doing that so often."

"I know Rebecca, but what are we supposed to do, turn them away? Let them suffer, or worse, die from simple things that I can cure?"

"You know I agree with you. However, we wouldn't be here at all without Mason Moose's funding."

"I know. This town didn't even have a proper doctor five years ago." Bryan rose as he spoke. "Speaking of which, I need to go have a word with Milly about following up with the Otters on her rounds. I'm worried they won't come back in for a checkup without a little nudge. I'll speak with Owl myself while I'm out."

"Good idea, Doctor. I'll hold down the fort until you get back."

* * *

As usual, the main street was abustle, animals going to and from businesses, working, shopping, or catching up on the latest gossip. Most of the townsfolk waved or smiled at Doctor Bison as he passed on his way to Owl's shop. A few stopped him to chat, but he excused himself quickly, knowing his own tendency to get caught up telling tales and chatting with every animal he ran into.

This was his town, his community. Just about every face he saw had been on his examination table or even on his operating table at one point or another over the past several years. He had delivered many of the children he saw playing along the main road.

This was his duty, his pride, and his passion.

Otis Owl ran the town's apothecary shop, which also doubled as a general goods store. The old place smelled of stringent herbs and soil.

"Afternoon, Bryan. Rebecca sent her boy over with today's scripts just a moment ago. What brings you by?" Otis swooped down from the rafter, landing behind the front counter.

Bryan greeted him with a smile. "Just needed to track down Milly about a few things and deliver the Otter's script personally. Go ahead and put them on my tab for the time being."

True to form, Otis fussed and fluffed up as he shuffled over to his ledger, all the while keeping silent. His plumage always gave him away.

"Just say it," Bryan coaxed.

"Oh, no no. Nothing to say. Not me. No, you're wise enough to know all on your own without my commentary. Besides, it's none of my business as long as the tab is settled at the end of the month." Owl twisted his head, peering up at the big bison upside down. The gesture was all too familiar to Bryan, a subtle jab from a longtime friend, and a warning.

"Don't worry yourself into a molt, Otis. Mason is a good fellow at heart. He'll see reason when need be."

"If anyone could convince a moose to live in a molehill, it's you, Doc. Oh, did—"

"I would love to stay and who's hoot all day with you Otis, but I've really got to be along before Milly heads back out to her hole for the evening."

"That joke never gets old, no sir," Owl drolled. "I was only going to let you know Milly came through here not an hour ago huffing and howling."

"What about?"

"Ol' Myron Mouse and his brood, you know. All come down with a fever, something fierce. She was headed out to the east fields when she left."

"Thank you, Otis. I'll head out there and see if I can't assist her."

* * *

The doctor was on the edge of town when a set of telltale antlers meandered out into the road ahead of him.

"Why Doctor Bison, what chance brings you along just when I was thinking of stopping by the office to see you?"

Bryan put on his most ingratiating smile. Mason Moose was not only his benefactor, but the richest creature in the territory. He was proud, haughty, and had a way of looking a lot farther down his already prominent nose at everyone. Still, Bryan generally got along with the fellow, if not going as far as to say he considered him a friend.

"I'll have to beg your pardon, Mister Mason, as I am on my way to see Milly."

"Hmm, I suppose it's late enough in the day to call it your own time to be venturing out of town?"

"You know I make house calls from time to time, Mason, when necessary."

"Of course. And I would never insinuate that you are anything but attentive to your patients. Even to a fault. Or rather, in this case, default."

"Sir?" Bryan could see where this was going, but he suppressed a grimace.

"Milly, being the town midwife and taking donations from the folk to see herself fed is one thing, Doctor. She has every prerogative to see to Myron Mouse at her leisure. I must, unfortunately, suggest that you let this one lie, as it were. The Mouses owe the practice for the last three visits."

"I see where you are coming from, Mason. However, the family is huge. He cannot possibly be accountable for every niece, uncle, and grandchild's visit to the infirmary. I will see to the bill getting properly delivered to the right party."

"Doctor, forgive me, but let me rephrase my statement. You are not to see the Mouses until they have settled their debt with us. Am I clear?"

Doctor Bison ground his teeth. He knew better than to let his temper lead him into locking horns to antlers with his boss. There were bigger battles than this to fight.

Or were there?

Was treating any patient, or not treating them, the most important fight of his life? Even at his own expense?

"You are very clear, sir. Now, if you'll excuse me, I am *off* for the day, and I would like to go see my friends, the Mouses."

Mason Moose's conciliatory nod told Bryan that the battle had truly only just begun.

Chapter Two

The Crowded Room

The Bison and the Weasel

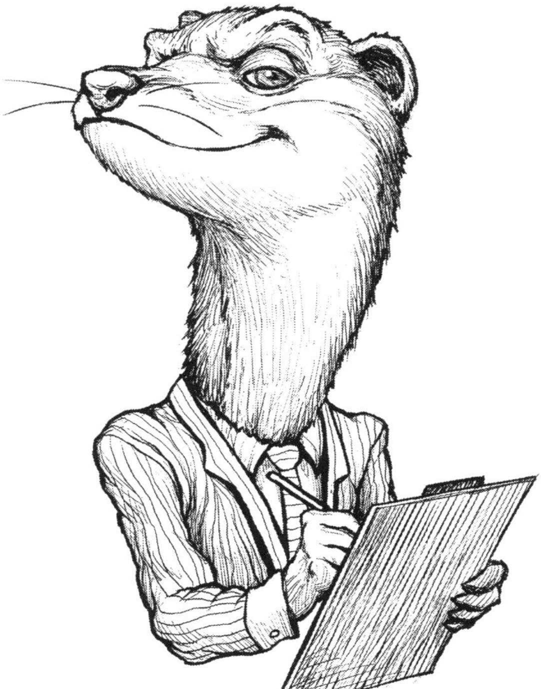

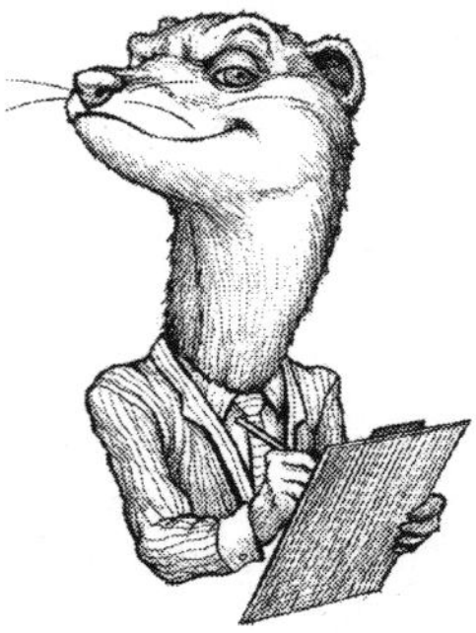

After many years of hard work, the bison found a place in a small community where he felt he could do some good. But the more the bison tried to help those in need, the more obstacles presented themselves.

One day, the bison came upon an injured duck and her ducklings. But before he could see to her damaged wing, the weasel emerged, giving him pause.

"Ah, good bison," the weasel said. "Would that I could let you help this poor mother?"

The bison knew that the weasel was a crafty and resourceful animal, so he asked, "What say do you have over whether I help her?"

"You see, this duck passed through my territory, and I have claimed them all under my protection. I cannot in good conscience allow her any other assistance but my own."

"But you are going to eat them, one by one," said the bison.

"Ah, you are correct. But they will each live a bit longer until I do, protected until I hunger again. Such is the nature of things. You are a bison; you cannot understand the way predators and prey work."

"You could eat one and let the others go."

"And leave me to starve in the future?"

Power uses safety and wellbeing as an excuse to control and regulate necessities.

EARLY MORNING SUNLIGHT POOLED on Doctor Bison's desk as he sat quietly, filling out sheet after sheet of paperwork. Mayor Weasel's newest rules mandated that he create new files for each patient with extensive history, all coded and organized for review. And it seemed like the system changed every day.

Who even needs to review all of this other than me or another doctor?

The past six months had seen a wave of new regulations placed on the townsfolk, all adamantly assured by the mayor to be for their benefit. Despite his misgivings, Bryan had to admit the town was thriving. Things seemed busier than ever.

However, for some reason, the majority of the new laws seemed to be geared toward scrutinizing his job and those of other specialized providers in the town. Owl had to hire two extra hands. Miss Gopher was having to do massive renovations to her tunnels for "proper and safe" storage procedures of the town's winter stores.

Mister Mason and the rest of the influential figures in town were conspicuously quiet on all the regulations.

"Just do what must be done, Bison. Better to play along with the mayor now, and get something we need later," Mister Mason told him when he brought up the insurmountable workload. "Choose your battles."

Shaking his head, Bison finished the file he was working on and stretched. His first patient would be arriving soon. At least he could focus on what really mattered, helping the injured and ill.

"Right this way, Mrs. Badger," Rebecca said as she ushered

the older animal into the examination room. Doctor Bison readied himself to smile and greet the familiar, but difficult, old badger.

He heard Rebecca say, "If you'd like to wait outside, sir?"

"No need, I'll be joining you," stated a gruff and throaty voice.

Doctor Bison hurried out of his office to see a surly, waddling beaver in a suit shoulder his way past Nurse Rabbit. The creature eyed the room from top to bottom, barely giving the doctor a second glance. He made several notes, frowning and shaking his head.

"Good morning, Mrs. Badger, get comfortable on the table there and I'll be right with you. And you are?" He turned back to the sour faced beaver.

"I'm never comfortable on your awful table," Mrs. Badger snipped. "And Mister Beaver is my attorney, Doctor. It has been brought to my attention that having someone around during dangerous situations like these is the wisest course."

"Dangerous situations?" Bryan asked, hesitantly taking the business card offered by the stout little lawyer.

"You take my life in your hands each and every time I visit this office. I am just taking precautions. The mayor says we all should. He's brought in all sorts of help to make sure everyone has access to proper protection."

The doctor and nurse exchanged exasperated looks, Nurse Rabbit shrugging slightly and shaking her head. Doctor Bison squared his shoulders and faced Mister Beaver.

"That's wonderful for everyone, to feel safer. But, for the sake of the comfort and privacy of my patient, I would prefer you wait outside, Mister Beaver. I'm sure Mrs. Badger can fill you in on anything you need to know, and you are welcome to review my paperwork after the appointment."

"It's precisely that sort of dismissive and careless behavior that I am here to prevent, Mr. Bison. You so-called health specialists have been without oversight for too long. Who knows what nonsense you convince people they're sick with?"

"It's Doctor. Doctor Bison. And I would never behave carelessly with my patients, sir. I only want what is best for any of them."

"Then you should have no issue with me watching you see to whatever Mrs. Badger *needs*. And *only* what she needs, mind you."

Bryan bit back a retort, gesturing for Mister Beaver to have a seat.

"Am I going to be made to wait all day, Doctor? I am old and in pain," Mrs. Badger shouted.

* * *

"This is outrageous!" Doctor Bison paced the room. He had to reschedule several patients in the wake of Mrs. Badger's excessively long appointment and follow up with Mister Beaver for questions. Even worse, two of the patients waiting in his lobby had brought attorneys of their own. There was no option though. Someone had to step in and fix this before it got out of hand.

Bryan just hoped that no emergency would come in while he was away.

"Agreed. You should have contacted me immediately, before seeing the patient." Mason Moose stood at the window of his spacious study gazing out over the lake.

"You're right," Bryan admitted. Best to let the boss give the order to get those nuisances out of his examination room.

Mr. Moose turned sharply. "We need to get one of my attorneys in there with you any time this happens. In fact, I would like to keep someone at the office from now on. Just for your protection, of course. Nip the whole thing in the bud."

Bison gaped. "I beg your pardon?"

"The only way to ensure that we are covered is to put our own securities in place. I have a feeling we will start to see this a lot more frequently, as the mayor encourages the townsfolk to protect themselves on every front. Good advice as far as I am concerned. I'll have someone there first thing tomorrow. They can also look over the paperwork you've been doing to make sure it meets all the regulations. This will also prevent the patients from having to wait so long. You cannot simply leave in the middle of the day like this either. I will check in more frequently as well, to make sure you have what you need."

Bryan staggered down the steps from Moose's mansion, his brain spinning. This was all absurd.

The walk back to town gave him time to think and organize his thoughts. Certainly, the mayor would see reason if he explained that these new rules were hindering him from helping the townsfolk. No one should have to wade through these deep waters to get medical aid. He just had to speak to Mayor Weasel face to face.

Perhaps no one had brought these things to his attention?

At the Mayor's office, several beavers bustled about on the bottom floor, stamping and filing, making notes and guiding various animals into different lines to wait. Doctor Bison approached the main desk and waited to be noticed. Finally, he cleared his throat.

"Yes?"

"I am here to see the mayor. I urgently need to speak with him."

"Do you have an appointment and the proper form?"

"No, but I am the town's doctor. This is a bit of an emergency."

"I see. Make sure you have your identification ready and take these forms for an emergency appointment and fill them out over there. When you are done, wait in *that* line, give them to the secretary and they will make sure you have the correct stamp to enter the queue for a meeting in the appropriate category."

"And then I can see the mayor?"

"Then you can receive a chit to return here at the earliest available date on which said topics are being addressed. After that, we will assign a time to see the mayor's aid so she can hear your reason for needing to speak with the mayor and decide the level of urgency."

"And let me guess, then you'll put me in a queue to schedule an appointment to get in line to wait and see if the mayor can get to me that day?"

"Precisely. I am relieved you know how it works already." The beaver smiled blandly, oblivious to the sarcasm.

By the time the doctor finished filling out the forms and waited in line, the sun was dipping low on the horizon. At least he was next in line, and he was one step closer to working all of this out. He would make sure he had a better way to contact the mayor in the future. They had always been on good terms in the past, and the town doctor *had* to be able to address urgent matters of public health.

"These are the wrong forms."

"Excuse me?"

"You have an emergency meeting form, but the information you filled out is for a rush appointment with the mayor over public health concerns. Please acquire the correct form and return it to us tomorrow during business hours." The teller window abruptly clacked shut.

Bryan's hoofs dragged through the dirt as he headed home, defeated. Maybe Mister Mason had a better way of getting in touch with the mayor. For now, he had to keep working, keep treating his community. What else could he do? And certainly, it would even out soon.

Things wouldn't get worse.

* * *

"Hold on a moment, Doctor. Nurse, does this patient have the proper card, proving they have paid for medical coverage?" The wiry ferret Mister Mason assigned to the Doctor's office had a shrill voice. In a little over a week, Mister Ferret had completely overhauled their system.

"I am not sure, ma'am," Rebecca said.

"Well, any patient must present their proof of coverage or pay up front before we can see them. Newest policy from the mayor's office. Tell the patient they will have to reschedule and let the Doctor know we are moving on to the next patient."

Chapter Three

Relating Too Well

The Bison and the Bull

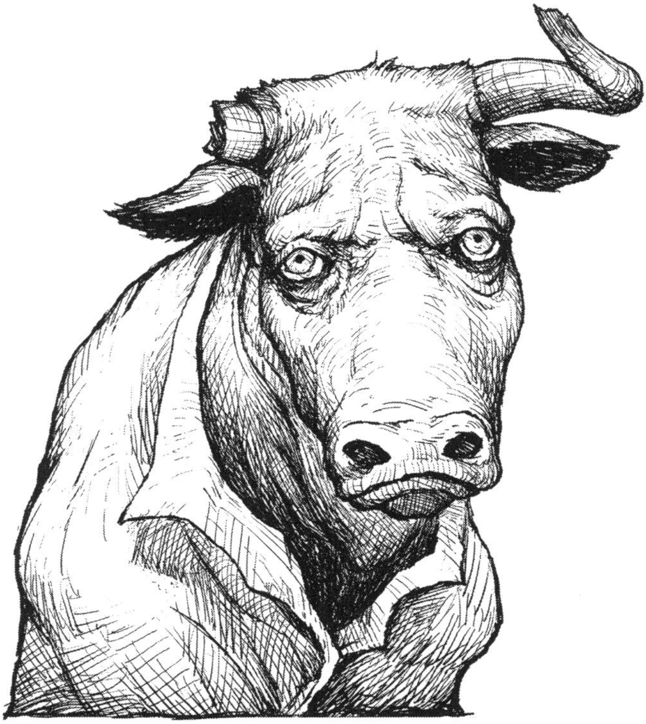

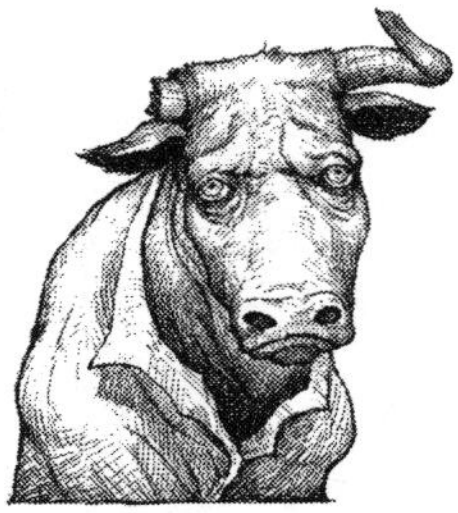

Late one evening, a bull came to the bison in pain. Although he clearly needed help, he was, being true to his nature, aggressive and demanding.

"Heal me. Take this pain away!" he shouted.

Despite the bull's manner, the bison saw the deep anguish of the bull's suffering. He knew pain all too well himself. So, he did what he could to alleviate the bruises, the broken horn. All the while, the bull complained and threatened the bison.

Soon, however, the bull rested.

The bison thought to himself, "I have done the right thing," and he retired for the evening.

In the morning, the bison found his home destroyed and the bull gone. The other animals who saw this said, "What a fool. He should have known what would happen."

"Regardless," the bison wondered, "How can I see someone so like me in need, and not help in any way I can?"

But in doing so, he put himself at great risk.

Caregivers must ride the line between relating and self-preservation.

THE LOUD NOISE CLATTERED AGAIN rousing Bryan from a deep sleep. His rooms above the clinic were still dark, but a hint of dawn colored the horizon out his window.

Another thump. Someone was downstairs.

Sometimes Nurse Rabbit came in early to clean or organize his office for the day. Or it could be an emergency patient, but the big bell outside hadn't rung. Suspicion drew him awake enough to rise, snatch his robe and slippers, and tiredly trek down the stairs to the door connecting his apartment to the offices.

As he entered, he tensed, noting the state of the back door. It was ajar, clearly scraped and splintered around the latch. Doctor Bison remained frozen to the spot, waiting. What should he do? He almost reached for the walking stick he kept in the pot by the door.

The clatter of clinking glass bottles reached him from the storeroom where they kept most of their supply of medicine, save for the very strong and dangerous concoctions locked in the basement. Weighing the risk, Bryan took a deep breath and pushed the door shut behind him, rather loudly. Simultaneously, he flicked on the lights in the hallway.

"If it's help you need, or some soothing for your woes, I'm sure there's something we can do." His offer hung in silence for several seconds. Hopefully, this trespasser was not debating whether to assault him as he dashed for the door.

"You can come out. I won't call the constable as long as we can have a talk. Tell me why you need whatever it is you're looking for in there."

Slowly, and somewhat menacingly, a large shadow shuffled out of the storeroom at the far end of the hall. There was still sufficient room between them that the doctor felt safe, the open door waiting if he needed to flee. The hunched figure stiffly turned, still imposing, but belying some insecurity.

Bryan felt the threat diminish palpably as he stared at the shivering creature. A trembling breath shuddered from the fellow's mouth as he looked up, shame and anger pasted all over his bovine face. "I-I'm sorry for b-breakin' in, mister. But you gotta give me something."

"Don't worry yourself. You look like you're in a lot of pain, friend." Bryan gestured toward the office door, keeping his movements slow and gentle. He was starting to recognize the symptoms. The bull, as he now could now make out, looked ragged, and someone had broken his horns off in the recent past. His clothes, once a working animal's overalls, were in tatters.

"Y-yessir. Hurts really bad. All over."

"Hmm. Have a seat and I'll put on some tea." Doctor Bison took the opportunity to circle the bedraggled bull, looking for signs of injury.

No obvious signs other than minor bruising, likely from the same fight where he lost his horn.

In the few minutes it took him to heat the water and steep some leaves, the doctor slipped into the storeroom and gathered a couple of jars of salve, unguents, and tools. He couldn't administer anything too heavy without knowing what the creature was on or had taken, that would risk a conflict of chemicals or adverse reaction.

"Here now, drink this and I will tend to those cuts and bruises."

"I said I just want somethin' for the pain," the bull growled, growing agitated.

"I understand, friend, and I will give you that, if you promise to let me take care of the rest. Can't have you getting an infection." Doctor B kept his voice soft but firm. The bull backed down, nodding his consent.

A pot of tea and several awkward, silent moments later, the bull's eyes were drooping from the mild sedative Bryan had brewed into the warm drink. The doctor guided the drowsing bull into the recovery room and sat him down on a cot.

"What's your name?"

A subdued glimmer of rage and pain flickered across the bull's face first, but then sorrow sagged his expression. How long had it been since anyone bothered to say a kind word or ask any courtesy of him?

"A-Abberdeen. Momma called me Abb." His eyes were glassing over a bit, his gaze distant.

"Well, Aberdeen, Abb. You stay here tonight. Get some rest. In the morning, I'll see that you're fed and send you along with a powder that will ease your aches. It will take some time to get better." Bryan had to fight the urge to preach to the fellow, to convey that if he continued to abuse whatever substance he was using, the pain would never go away. The only thing that would really make much of a difference would be to show kindness, offer stability, and tangible assistance in the form of food and rest and send the creature on its way.

For now.

If he could become a safe haven for those who sought succor, eventually some might return, seeking a more permanent solution and treatment. This was something very near to Bryan's heart, to heal those with the deepest pain, those who had been shunned by society and the community and who would not, or could not, find a way back. Reaching those individuals was one of the main reasons he got into medicine, and as things go, unfortunately was one of the hardest things to find the time and resources for. Mister Mason, for one, was far from interested in spending time or funding for such endeavors.

By now, the sun had peaked over the hills, announcing the start of the working day for the community.

True to form, Nurse Rabbit came bustling in, shooing the doctor back upstairs to get dressed and eat something proper prior to the long day of visits he had on the books. She paused after a glance into the recovery room and gave the doctor a stern look. “Doctor B, Mister Ferret will be here shortly. Are you sure we shouldn’t send that poor chap on his way before he does? I know full well he isn’t a paying customer, or someone who could afford the mayor’s coverage. And I know too well your heart on the matter.”

The *but* hung in the air as Doctor Bison frowned, pausing at the stairs. Every excuse and response he had was moot. Nurse Rabbit held all his same beliefs on taking care of those who needed it. But she had a way of being far more rational and realistic, especially given their current situation and oversight. “He’ll just have to understand. And I’ll make sure it’s clear that this was on me, out of pocket. He’ll be moving along soon enough.”

An hour later, Doctor B squinted, looking through the scope into the long fuzzy ears. “I can get the buildup out today, Jack, but you’re going to need to clean your ears a bit more regularly to avoid this happening again, alright?”

“Sure thing, boss, sure indeed,” Jack Hare agreed, stopping mid nod.

A soft chuckle escaped the doctor’s muzzle. “Careful there. Hold extra still.”

Out of the corner of his eye, Doctor Bison caught movement in the hall. Mister Ferret was doing his rounds with his clipboard, checking everything in the building like he did every day. His first stop was always the storeroom for stock, next he would undoubtedly check the recovery room since the door was closed. He could feel the beady little glare from the doorway, waiting for him to turn and acknowledge him. "With a patient. Be done soon," he muttered casually.

The next patient and one more kept the pest at bay until just before lunch, as Mrs. Goat fussed into the office, throwing a fit about her swollen udders. Mister Ferret stepped out to block Bryan's way before he entered the exam room.

"Doctor, I realize you are preoccupied and quite busy. However, it is my purview to note any and all comings and goings, material and usage. I must have the forms for the medicine that is missing from the cabinet," he hesitated, nodding overtly toward the back room. "Is that an unscheduled patient, with no records or identification receiving special treatment and a free bed?" Exasperated, his voice choked off in a shrill whistle at the end.

"I was going to discuss it with you after the morning rush," Bison began when a harsh bleat interrupted them from the examination room.

"What's this I hear? Rest in a private room? Special medications? Why have I not been offered such a remedy, Doctor? I can hardly get enough sleep to get well at home, and you've never bothered to give me that option. I knew there must be something better you could give me for this."

"Mrs. Goat, what you need is to stay active, work on the diet we discussed last time, and take the anti-inflammatories I prescribed. The recovery room is for special cases and for after surgery."

For once, Mister Ferret backed him up, nodding in agreement. Of course, he would support not using any resources unnecessarily.

"So, I am not worth it, is that it? What an outrage. Some vagrant can waltz in here and get the good stuff and us working folk are left with good wishes and a slap on the wrist for eating what we enjoy."

Doctor B bit his tongue. *The food you enjoy is what is causing most of your issues.* He resisted the urge to say, "I promise you are getting the care you need, Margaret—"

"Nonsense. The Mayor and Mister Mason will be hearing about this travesty. We'll see if you are peddling your snake oil for much longer, you crook." She baa-ed as she stormed out, her small hoofs rat-a-tatting on the floor.

"Hmm. You could have handled that better," Mister Ferret grumbled, shaking his head. "I'll have to write you up for poor customer interaction. Now, regarding your negligent use of medicines—"

"Negligent? I only gave the poor fellow a mild sedative and some tincture to help him sleep off his inebriation."

"Precisely. I found the containers in your office. Which means you allowed that vagabond to steal from us. Negligence. Carelessness. I should have searched him."

"What do you mean? Where is he?" He only just now noticed the room was empty.

"I sent him packing, of course. This isn't a hostel or a boarding house, Doctor."

"But I told him we would give him something to eat. If we kick him out, he will just go try to find something to kill the pain he is in."

"Sounds like a ne'er-do-well, indeed. Good thing I got rid of him. The constable will make sure he moves on. You are lucky he didn't cause any further trouble. You'd be culpable."

"Still, I promised him more."

"Well then, it sounds like you should not make promises you cannot keep to customers who cannot pay."

"Customers?" Doctor Bison felt the first pangs of fear for his calling as the word lingered in the air. Anger and regret welled up, railing at the unfairness, while he felt mad at himself for caring so much, for trying to do the right thing. For the first time in his life, he wondered if what he was doing was worth it.

Chapter Four

Fear and Superstition

The Bison and the Crow

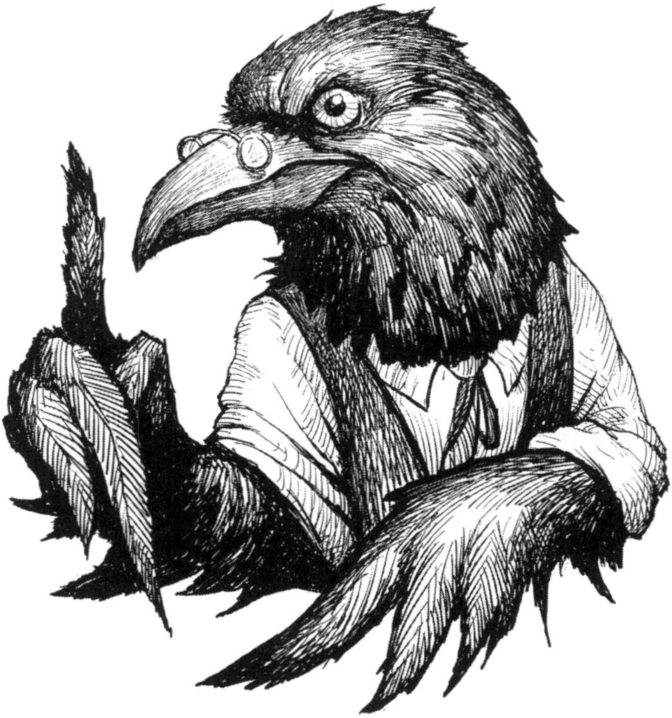

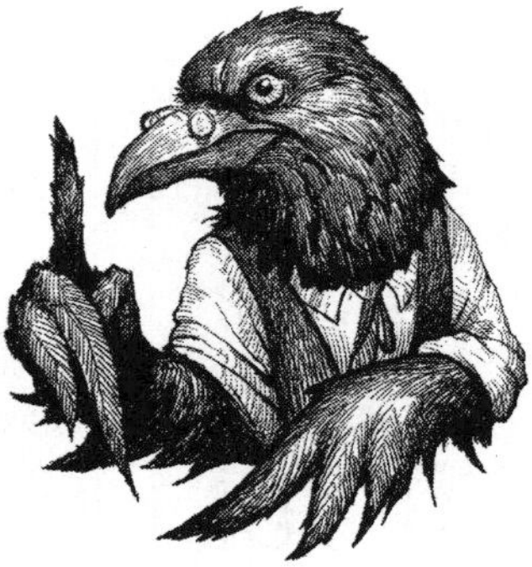

Now the crow, being a suspicious and crafty creature, assumed that every other animal was out to take advantage of him. After all, each and every animal had to fend and fight for itself to get what it needed, same as he.

So it was, when the crow needed help with a troublesome and irritating burr in his feathers that he couldn't reach with his beak, he made his way to the bison, who he knew to be a helpful and learned creature. Surely, he would help the crow, albeit for his own motives and gain, but the crow would be careful not to be taken for a fool.

The bison quickly assessed the matter, and with a quick flick, had the burr removed from the delicate down feathers near the crow's skin. Though the bison had been gentle and removed it swiftly, the crow shrieked as if in agony.

"Ouch! You've hurt me with your rough treatment. I thought you were supposed to be a healer," cawed the crow. "I'm worse off now than if I had suffered the minor inconvenience of the burr."

And all the animals of the community saw this and looked at the bison warily, even though they had known him for years.

With great responsibility comes ever greater accountability, but accountability can quickly turn to blame.

"THIS IS OUTRAGEOUS. Do you know how much I have already paid just to ensure the right to come see you and be protected from illness?" Mister Crow puffed his feathers fitfully, pacing the examination room.

"I understand, Emmet, but the treatment is vital for your recovery. Between medicines, materials, and my time, these things have to cost something. I am sorry for the inconvenience. If you have issues with the security or the pricing, you should bring it to the mayor's attention." Doctor Bison tried as hard as he could to keep his tone congenial and pleasant, even if he felt anything but.

Or he could try nagging Mister Mason for bankrolling this terrible system.

The frequency with which his patients were becoming agitated with the new system was wearing him down. Or rather, the way they criticized and complained about his doctoring, as if any of it were his doing.

He knew, however, that being the face they saw and the only one they had access to, made him the most likely subject on whom to take out their frustrations. Unlike the faceless providers of this new service, he could not limit his patients' access to him or his treatment if they were to heal.

Or could he?

An imminent future was looming where doctors might have to do that very thing. And what a bleak future that would be. But the more he thought about it, the more certain he was that the best way to safeguard against the growing unrest and possible danger to his career would be to bottleneck the patient-doctor interaction. Just like how the insurers placed steps upon steps of regulation to offer coverage for medical expenses, the doctor could minimize contact and liability by delegating more tasks to nurses, creating diversions to shuffle minor issues to less qualified healers, balancing risk to ability.

And in doing so, he thought. *We would remove the most important thing about healing. Remove the care from caregiving.*

In his own heart, Bryan struggled with a growing anger and frustration, fueled by the worry, stress, and fear for his patients and his own wellbeing. He had half a mind to force his way into the mayor's office to let him have it. Not to mention Mister Mason, who he'd only contacted through his representative in the office in recent weeks.

It was like they only cared about the money and putting every conceivable roadblock in the way of anyone receiving the care they needed. To top things off, someone always laid the blame at his hoofs, as if he had facilitated and encouraged this chaos.

And explaining all of that to his patients was foolish, he knew. They did not care about the semantics of who was truly to blame for their struggles. They just wanted and/or needed those hurdles to go away, to stop feeling like they were being scammed.

A scam is surely what it was, and it got worse with each passing month. Already, he was inundated with paperwork, fees, signatures, and duplicates. Even with the new assistant nurse he had brought on and Mr. Ferret's secretary, Miss Vole, the workload of documentation alone was inhibiting their capacity to see everyone who tried to get an appointment.

Doctor Bison shook his head, jogging his mind back to the present. "I'll do what I can to keep the cost as low as I can for you, Emmet."

"Simple thievery is what this all is. I know you are just trying to do your job, Doctor. You've always done right by us, and I appreciate you," Mister Goose conceded as Nurse Rabbit ushered the elder from the room, quietly instructing him how to properly check out with the front desk and how to set up the appointment for the therapy sessions if he should decide to get them.

What a concept, considering not going through with a very necessary and helpful series of treatments to alleviate the damage from his torn wing muscle.

Yet, that's what it had come to. More and more often, his patients opted to just deal with the pain, shrugging that they couldn't afford it, or the hoops they would have to jump through to try to get it covered weren't worth the time and effort. These were simple animals who had lives, families, and jobs, and hardly the time to spend arguing with someone in an office over getting better and moving on with what they had to do.

Even the wealthier creatures with better coverage still quibbled and squabbled over the details. In many cases they failed to complete their treatment regimen before they defaulted on their monthly payment, or some new rule came along that no longer covered the cost.

In the best cases, the system seemed to keep things running, but as it grew more and more complex to address every issue that arose, he understood it less and less. How could anyone keep up?

The apothecary, Mister Owl, was up in arms over it as well, trying to keep up with the almost daily shifts in who he could sell medicine to, what type they qualified for, and how he was to source all of it.

Doctor Bison washed thoroughly before hanging his coat on the rack. He had a bit of time before his next appointment. A bit of fresh air would serve him well. As he stepped out the back door, he felt sad relief. It used to be difficult to take breaks. Now he was beginning to hate being in that office, eager for the next chance he would have to leave for even a temporary reprieve.

A short walk later, he found himself by the creek, musty scents and a cool breeze soothing his stress and frustration. Perhaps this could be a way for him to manage, taking more frequent breaks. Something had to give.

Unfortunately, the little voice in the back of his head argued the flaw in that reasoning. Having to come up with bandages and stop-gaps to tolerate the way things were would only last so long. It would be too much like a strong pain-relieving pill that dealt with short-term symptoms of a chronic ailment.

With a deep sigh, Bryan turned and headed back to the office. He couldn't stay away too long, and he needed to check in with Mister Owl about a few things before the workday finished.

No sooner had he crossed the edge of the outlying buildings near his home than a small critter came bounding up to him, looking frazzled.

"Doc, Doc!" the young otter shouted, catching his breath.

"Philip, what's the matter?"

"It's Miss Milly Mole, sir. She was out at our place giving my lil' sister a checkup when they came pounding on the door."

"Who, Philip?"

"Some fancy dressed fellows. They said she had to leave and come with them."

A thousand thoughts rushed through the doctor's head. Who would go to trouble to follow Milly all the way out to the Otters on her rounds? And who did they think they were to order her to cease her duties? There was more to the situation, certainly, but Philip, as eager as he seemed to help, would not have the answers.

"Okay, Philip. First, was everyone alright at your house?"

"Yes, Doc. Momma said Miss Milly told her Christy will be fine. It's just a cough."

"Good. Next, do you know where Miss Milly was taken after she left?"

"Yessir. They took her to the courthouse straight away. Pa and me followed them back to town before he sent me to get you. He was shoutin' something fierce at them, Pa was."

"Well, let's hope your dad didn't get himself into any trouble, too." Doctor Bison ushered the little otter along down the street. None of this made sense. Milly had been the town's midwife for nearly thirty years and was beloved by everyone she met. There were few families that didn't have her to thank for most of their children and grandchildren being safely delivered.

A sour feeling started in his gut as they rounded the corner onto the main thoroughfare leading to the town hall. And it was more than just his own uncertainty and unease with the current climate of health-related affairs. There was a general tension in the town among the people he had come to cherish and care for. Every face showed worry and a distant gaze.

They were scared. Stressed.

When had things gotten so bad? In the months since the Mayor and Mason had implemented new regulations, it seemed the town had undergone a transformation. More than the growing populace, the way everyone seemed to be working longer hours and spending less time recuperating and relaxing was changing the culture of their small community.

"Thank heavens, Doc. You gotta do something," Philip Otter, Senior stopped his pacing as soon as he caught sight of the odd pair approaching. "I tried to tell them they couldn't do it, but they locked her up. Then they threatened the same for me if I didn't move along, as I have no relation to Miss Milly. As if we all aren't part of her family."

Bryan shook his head, unsure what to say in response. This entire situation was so out of control, out of character from the town he knew. It was unbelievable.

"Mister Otter, I'll see what I can do. Just keep calm, and don't cause a scene. The last thing we need is to escalate this whole business and get you in trouble. And seeing as how I am a colleague, maybe I can get some answers."

The deep-seated unrest burned off as anger and outrage took its place. He had about enough of this mess. Bryan squared his shoulders and stomped into the town hall.

Chapter Five

Held Hostage

The Coyote and the Bison

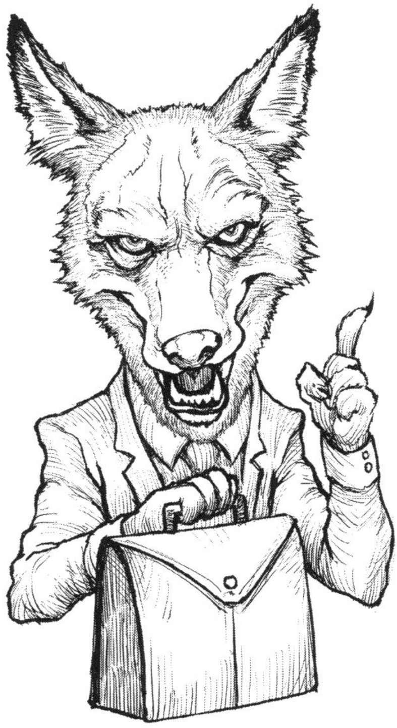

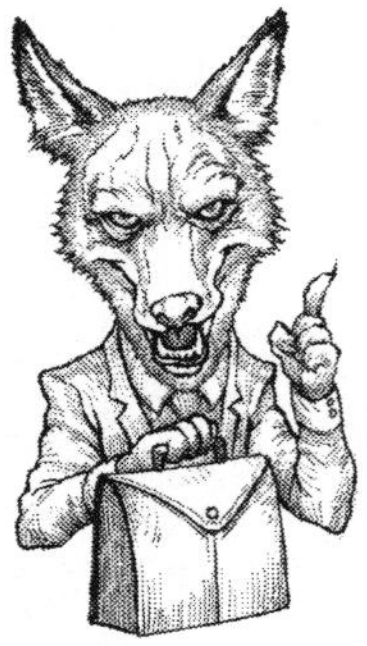

As time passed, new predators moved into the territory, claiming it as their own. The threat caused an increase in visitors to the bison, both for fear of attack and injuries.

One day, another animal came running to tell the bison that his friend, the owl, was caught in a thicket. So, the bison rushed to assist him. In the owl's panic, he called out, and so too came the coyote, hearing the sound of helpless prey.

"Leave him be, coyote," said the bison.

"But why, when I am here to help? I can more easily pull him from the thicket than you."

"Ouch!" cried the owl. The bison paused his ministrations, worrying about hurting his friend.

"Move aside, bison," said the coyote, licking his chops.

"No. I do not trust you. You will hurt him more, or worse."

So, the bison pulled the owl from the thicket. In the tangle, the owl's wing caught, and a bone broke as the bison tugged him free. The bison hurried to set the bone and wrapped the appendage.

When other animals came near to see what the commotion was, the coyote warned them off. "Be careful, the bison might trample you, then offer to heal you for a price."

"I would not do such a thing," protested the bison.

"But do you not take advantage of every creature's injury, holding their health hostage with your knowledge?"

"I have sworn to help those in need. I do not cause that need."

"But when I offered to help, you refused to let me, even though I might have saved the poor creature from a broken limb," the coyote argued.

"I was trying to protect my friend from you, a known predator."

But the other animals grew more fearful in the predator's presence and turned angry gazes on the bison. "We must protect ourselves from you."

And so, the bison was chased from the community, not by the pack of coyotes, but by the animals he had sworn to heal.

The culture of fear turns victims against those that can help them.

"THE CASE IS QUITE SIMPLE, YOUR HONOR. There are rules in place for the safety of medical patients. They guard innocent people from the failures of negligent caregivers." The slender coyote turned as he spoke, pointedly looking toward the frazzled mole seated behind the defendant's desk. "Unauthorized practice of medicine cannot go unaddressed. There are clear definitions of safe measures, proper procedure, and licensing. Miss Mole stated herself, that she followed none of these. She maliciously misled patients into thinking she was qualified to treat them."

"But the system is so convoluted that no one could possibly be expected to keep up," Mother Mole stuttered. "I have served this town as midwife for three decades—"

"The defendant will not speak out of turn," Judge Falcon snapped, clacking his beak for order.

Counselor Coyote seized his advantage. "Thank you, your honor. But she brings up a valid point. Those who serve in the system must be able to understand and follow it. Those who cannot, have no place conducting complex and dangerous procedures on unsuspecting patients. Further, by her own admission, she has done so recklessly for, how long did you say Miss Mole? Thirty years? I move that the sentence be compounded to reflect that time-frame."

"Objection, your honor, the system has only been in place for a year." Counselor Woodchuck glared at his counterpart. The case was not going well for the defense.

"Overruled. Does the prosecution have evidence of previous malpractice?"

"Indeed, your honor. We have hundreds of accounts from interviews conducted with dozens of townsfolk documenting her extensive history of medical fraud dating back thirty-two years, including events performed while underage." Coyote sneered.

The packed courtroom erupted in murmurs and shocked gasps of denial. Nearly every animal present looked horrified by the revelation that their unwitting testimonies were now being used against the poor midwife.

"We thought we were helping explain."

"If I would have known they would turn it on her."

"She delivered my baby. Of course, I told them."

"Order!" Judge Falcon shouted over the commotion. "The trial will be closed to the town if the audience cannot remain silent."

The crowd's chatter abated. In the ominous quiet that settled, Coyote cleared his throat with a growl of feigned remorse. "Distressing indeed. As I was saying, while underage—"

Mother Mole's voice rose, trembling in protest. "Your honor, please, I apprenticed with my mother when I was girl. That hardly—"

"Defense, please communicate the severity of speaking out to your client. I will hold her in contempt if she continues to interrupt."

"Yes, your honor." Counselor Woodchuck patted Milly's hand reassuringly.

"Call your next witness, counselor."

"The prosecution calls Doctor Bryan Bison to the stand." More murmuring followed, this time much more subdued and far less concerned. The town trusted the doctor and seemed to have faith that he would be able to see something done to right this injustice.

And let's hope that I can, thought Doctor Bison.

After taking the oath and making his way to the podium, the doctor took a deep breath. He could almost feel the coyote licking his chops as he sorted through his paperwork on the desk, clearly drawing out the tension on purpose. Finally, he stood and sauntered to the center of the speaking floor. "State your position and credentials for the court, please."

"I am a physician. A medical doctor." He had rehearsed some of his responses with Nurse Rabbit the night before, practicing at keeping his answers as short and concise as possible. Doctor B knew himself too well, and his propensity for getting carried away with informative explanations.

"How long have you known the defendant, Doctor?"

"We have worked together for several years, since I returned to town and started my practice."

"And during that time, has the defendant worked for your office?"

"Um, no. She is independent of my practice." Bryan could see the way the questioning was heading but could not see how to divert his answers.

"A practice that is fully legal and licensed, correct?"

"Yes."

"And this is your license?" The coyote held up a copy of the document for the room to see.

"Yes."

"And do you know if the defendant, Miss Mole, has one of these, herself?"

A sickening feeling washed over the doctor. "No, I do not believe she does."

"Hmm. So she is, in fact, unlicensed."

"Be that as it may, she is as experienced as any doctor—"

"That is irrelevant. If she is as experienced as you say, she could, then go and get the necessary credentials and proper documentation with little effort."

"Objection, your honor—" Mister Woodchuck stood.

"Speculation. Sustained."

"Withdrawn, your honor. However, the fact remains that she has not attended medical school."

Dr. Bison quietly interjected, "If I may, your honor, I have learned as much from Mother Milly about practical medicine as I ever did in school. She is a healer by trade if not education, and a good one. Any member of our community would agree with me."

"This trial is not about what the community thinks of Miss Mole, Doctor. It is about the law. Counselor, any further questions?" Judge Falcon waved for Coyote to continue.

"By your own admission Doctor, you are licensed under the current legal system, yet you condone Miss Mole's activities. By that logic, anyone here, myself included, should be able to see to the needs of your patients."

"That is ridiculous."

"So, you are saying an unlicensed person should not practice medicine?"

"No. She is trained—"

"By you?"

"No."

"By the board of medicine?"

"*No.*"

"So, she is doing something illegal?"

"Yes. Technically." Bryan's shoulders slumped with defeat. "But I've overseen all the work she did since I have been here—made sure it was safe," he offered.

"Doctor, are you saying that you frequently delegate your duties as the town's doctor to someone else?"

The implication drew the doctor up short.

"I am not on trial here," Bryan stated through gritted teeth.

"Not yet." The coyote smirked as he returned to his desk. "No further questions."

"It's this system that should be on tri—" Bryan stood abruptly. He had to say something to stop this travesty.

Motion in the back of the courtroom caught his eye, and Bryan stopped short. Mister Mason was standing, shaking his head subtly but sternly, his horns jerking side to side. The message was clear.

Doctor Bison felt another stab of guilt and anger. So much of this rested on Mason's shoulders, and no one was calling on him, accusing him of anything. Worst of all, Bryan was complicit by working for the tycoon.

"Court adjourned until tomorrow at 9AM," the judge announced as he flapped down from the podium.

Doctor Bison stood on shaky legs, stumbling from the stand in a daze. Milly had been his friend and colleague for years. She had taught him so many methods and techniques, practical experience from an active caregiver they couldn't teach in medical school.

Outside, the bustle of the dispersing crowd blurred around him. Folks asked him questions he didn't hear. He just needed to get away, clear his head.

But the questions wouldn't let him go, not when he tried to sleep. Not when he tried to work. Not when the guilty verdict came back a few days later, sentencing Miss Milly to jail time and fines.

What could he have said differently? How could he have prevented this? The past year had washed by in a flood of change, a veritable bureaucratic mudslide. And he hadn't had a chance to even get a handle on it in his own life, his own work.

How long would it be until he was the one on trial?

The weeks that followed faded together. A rush of scared patients. Everyone was eager to speak with him, not only to ensure they were properly taken care of and up-to-date with the new system, but also to hear his take on the situation.

Surely, being the expert on such matters, he would have answers to their concerns. But as each day passed, distrust grew. Bryan didn't have the answers. He did his best to calm them. He tried to explain as best he could. More often than not, he had to defer them to Mister Ferret, both for a lack of time and a lack of knowledge about every new detail and rule.

Sometimes, he just didn't want to give them answers. Frankly, he thought, I am just terrified that one of them will take what I say and use it against me.

* * *

Doctor B trudged through the rain and into Otis Owl's shop. He hadn't been by in quite some time to see his friend, but today's visit was not a social call.

"Bryan, how's the day findin' you? Spot of rain to settle the dust."

Otis's usual chipper banter felt forced, strained.

"Things are definitely coming down out there, Otis." Bryan couldn't resist a wry smile, trying to coax and calm the tension that was hanging between them. Owl had made an odd habit lately of canceling or refusing to fill some of his patients' scripts. He finally had the time and the nerve to come find out why.

"Well, if you don't need anything, I best be getting back to it."

"We both know why I am here, Otis."

"Look here, Doc, I don't want to squabble with you. Just trying to do my job and keep things on the up and up, you know."

"Oh, I know. And I know you've been scared since Milly's trial. You've barely spoken to me." Bryan didn't bother to hide the hurt in his voice, the worry.

"What's there to speak about? Too much to do, not enough time."

"But that's just it. You haven't been doing much of anything when it comes to my prescriptions."

"They—"

"I understand. I'll leave you be, but please, at least fill Tom's refill for pain medication. For me."

"Honestly, Doc, I don't feel comfortable giving that fellow more drugs."

Bryan nearly scoffed. "Well, it's not for *your* comfort, is it, Otis? It's for the patient's comfort."

Otis fluffed up his feathers, his eyes darting every which way. It was time for the doctor to leave. The owl followed him out to lock up for the day, but just before he slammed the door, he hesitated, pulling the door open just a crack to say, "Doc, be careful. I've already been fined. They threatened to shut me down. They'll be coming for you next."

Sure enough, the very next day, a coyote was in his office when the doctor returned from a house call.

"Doctor Bison. This is a notice suspending your medical license pending investigation."

Chapter Six

Breeding Resentment

The Bison and the Viper

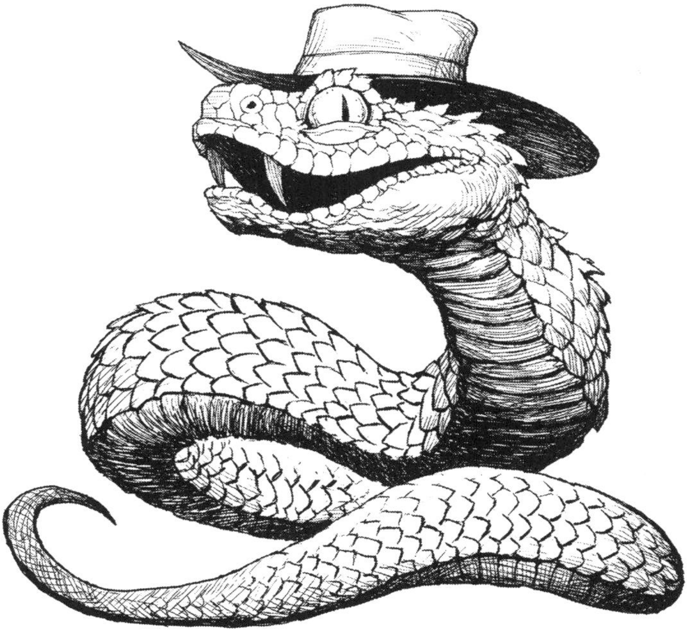

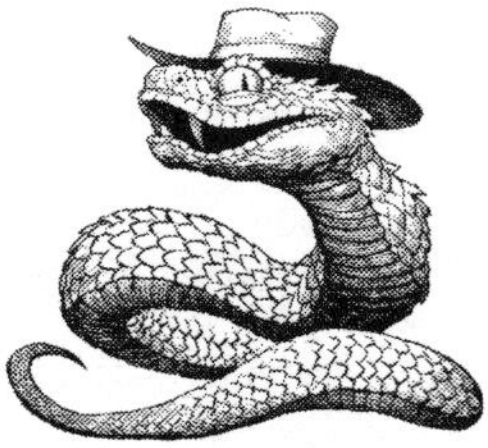

The bison roamed across the land, at times assisting those in need. Other times, he hid his nature and his abilities, conflicted by his right to intervene. Most often, he found that he selfishly did not want to risk his own safety simply for the sake of his old convictions.

One day, while journeying through a ravine, the bison found his path blocked by a large stone. As he approached, he heard a hiss and a crackling warning of a viper's tail rattle. Assessing the situation, the bison noticed that the viper was trapped by the stone.

Now, in the animal world, it is well known that the viper is a dangerous creature, but mostly just when threatened or cornered. The same can be said of many animals, but the viper in particular, being extremely deadly, is treated as a villain.

"You there, large creature," the viper hissed. "If you shove this rock aside with your strength, I will be free and let you pass."

Despite its claims, the bison knew that if he helped the viper, he would likely get bitten out of reflex. However, if he ignored it and let it die, would he be guilty of treating the snake as a villain as he had been treated?

The bison fought with himself for hours, finally reaching a decision. He would do what he could to help the snake and stay true to his beliefs.

But the snake was already dead.

Conviction is a double-edged sword: it can drive righteous motives forward, or it can lead to ultimatums and inaction.

* * *

BRYAN STOOD OVERLOOKING THE VASTNESS of the plains. It seemed endless, vacant, empty, but pristine. How could something so beautiful feel so meaningless to him?

A hollowness filled his soul where his calling had once resided.

In contrast, with all the righteous fury in his heart, he was far from empty. He was full of anger, sadness, and regret. The aftershock of the emotional fallout of his decision, not to mention the actual physical change that had come along with it, had not yet settled as a reality.

It was hard to believe only two weeks ago, his life had been normal, albeit miserable. Now he lingered in a limbo of doubt and uncertainty, not unlike the shaky ground he was treading in his practice—or rather, the ground he was treading before he quit—before he confronted Mister Mason, lost his cool, and made a rash decision.

"How could you allow this to happen, Mason? We set out to help people. Your funding was supposed to—" The words burst from him before he was even through the door of Mason's office.

"To make me money, Bryan. And yes, to help people. Ultimately. You can't say it didn't benefit you, too."

"I never took advantage of anyone. Nor was I consulted on how this disastrous system of insurance should even work."

"That's what accountants are for Bryan. Someone must

handle the money side of everything. And there is a money side to everything."

"More like ransom for helping innocent folk."

"You know better than most that there must be regulations in place to guarantee the safety of both the patients and the caregivers. Remember back when we were young? How many myths and superstitions surrounded medical treatments? It's a wonder we survived the leeches or infections."

Doctor Bison shook his head. He would not be diverted by anecdotes or platitudes. "That just means it's getting better. And we must be better, too."

"And what am I to do? Give away the product of my investment? The mayor's plan fell in line with my goals, and it was the only option presented to guide medical progress." Mason shrugged and lit a cigar, motioning for Bryan to sit.

He refused, wafting the poisonous smoke away with his hoof.

Mason continued, "Frankly, it's done more good than bad. How many more patients have you seen since this started? Members of the community who would never have had access to the service you provide are coming into town not only to meet their medical needs, but purchasing other goods as well."

"I like how you carefully omitted the fact that it is bankrupting those same poorer patients."

"It costs money to live. I guess we should let them die then. But then there would be no business at all."

Bison snorted, "and that your other businesses are booming as a result. How convenient. When the factory opens by the river, will you force all the employees you're bringing in to sign up as well? To give the money you pay them back to you for wellbeing?"

"I never claimed to be anything but a business moose, Doctor.

And yes, I have designs for an amended plan, with the mayor's approval, or at least, he will approve it if he knows what is good for his town. It will be incorporated into their pay scale, along with many other benefits we have never before been able to offer the working class. This is progress, Doctor."

"It's . . . it's robbery. There's something fundamentally wrong with it, Mason."

"What's wrong is your attitude and your performance. That outburst in court. You represent not only yourself and your practice, Bryan, but you also represent me. You'd do well to take better care in what you say to folks about any of this. Miss Mole suffered a sad fate. Mister Owl is soon to follow if he can't settle with the company over his infractions. I don't want you to be the next one on the block. I've already taken steps to get your suspension lifted."

"You don't have to worry about that. I won't stand for this any longer. I've already been threatened and controlled. My friends and colleagues have been run out of town, fined, jailed. I will not be next."

"What are you saying?"

"I'm saying that they can't sue me or come after my practice if I don't have one. I quit. Find another doctor who will play your games."

No longer would he stand by while Mister Mason and Mayor Weasel drove his patients against him, and corrupted what should be a most sacred relationship between a caregiver and his patient. A hopelessness threatened on the edge of those thoughts that he would never be a doctor again. That his protests would make no difference.

The growing wall of despair wobbled behind him, following him out of town before first light that next morning. It rushed like a storm across the plains, chasing him. But the doctor would not be crushed under its weight. He wanted to push back, to fight. Instead, he would push onward, away from it.

Nurse Rebecca begged him to stay. Thankfully, few others got wind of his departure.

Bryan crested another rise, the sun rushing toward the horizon. He would stop for the night soon, make camp. Sleep. Having simple and necessary things to occupy him helped. Gave him a purpose.

For now however, he knew he had to face that shadow within him, both the ache of abandoning his post, and the reality of the situation in his hometown. He just needed time to think and figure out how to go about fixing the problem.

I will find a better way, he thought. He just wished he could convince the pit in his stomach that he wasn't just making excuses or running away.

A few days later found the road-weathered doctor coming upon dryer, more rocky terrain, mesas, and ravines. This was the path he had chosen, to go west rather than east, for the only thing that waited back that way was the city where he had studied, and likely more legal problems.

Instead, he wandered into the open spaces where he knew he could doctor those truly in need. Perhaps he could find that spark again, of really offering wellness to those who had no access to healthcare. At least he would be useful.

Yet, several times along the road, Bryan avoided those very situations. The family of migrant goats he passed in his first week on the road could have used his advice and simple tips on hygiene and cleanliness. Their surliness and distrust of outsiders made it all too easy to move along and ignore them.

At the river crossing, an elderly beaver with a lame foot begged for change and food. Although Bryan shared the loaf of bread he had with him, the afternoon ferry was leaving. He used the excuse that he was in a hurry and couldn't miss it to explain his neglect of the infection spreading through the creature's bad paw.

Of course, he felt ashamed. But the general mood in some of the locales he passed through was often unfriendly, if not hostile. Marauding bandits were frequent occurrences in some of the villages along the main trail. Outsiders were held up and robbed and just as often killed. He knew he had to be wise and shouldn't draw too much attention to himself.

Then why am I out here?

Coward.

"Rocks fell through the canyon. Looks like we have to take the long way around."

Bryan perked up, the voices carrying back to him through the dust of the scrublands. A wagon took shape ahead, surrounded by a small group of animals of various species. They all looked road weary and filthy. These were hard living folk, laborers, possibly pioneers. Or possibly bandits.

"Pardon, but I overheard what you said. How long is the way around?" Bryan did his best to appear unassuming. They had surely spotted him on the road before he noticed them. He only hoped they hadn't stopped here as a trap to rob him.

The wiry bobcat scout eyed him up and down, his eye flinching suspiciously. Even after weeks on the road, the doctor stood out. He was a town creature.

"Three days south. Going to set us back."

"And that's the only way?"

"A lone traveler could climb through the canyon with the right gear. But we can't leave the wagons with all our wares, or what's the point?"

"Would you fine gentlemen happen to know where a lone

traveler might acquire the right gear to pass through the canyon?"

* * *

Treating the myriad of travel-related ailments only took the rest of the morning. Bryan disinfected cuts, set a dislocated shoulder, a broken paw, and cleaned and bandaged dozens of blisters. All in trade for a pack full of food, rope, and anything else the team thought he might need. After insisting he stay to share their lunch, he made good time with their directions into the canyon.

Four hours later, he came upon the rockslide. With little effort he scaled it using the hook and rope. The weeks of walking helped him get into fair shape.

As he lowered himself down near a large boulder on the far side, he froze to the sound of a sharp rattle.

Bill Bobcat was forthcoming with a slew of good advice once they had broken bread together. "Watch out for pebbles rolling. Keep aware of flash flooding. And most important, watch out for vipers. You'll only get one warning."

Slow and steady, thought the bison. The sound came from behind a rock formation.

He leaned out and hopped off the rockslide in the opposite direction when the rattle sounded again. Against his better judgment, he turned to peer around the large boulder. There, crushed under the huge rock, was a rattlesnake.

His training took him a step forward to ascertain whether the creature could be saved. Instinct kicked in a second later, drawing him up short. The creature wasn't moving. From where he stood, the doctor could see some blood, and the size of the rock made his choice for him.

The creature could not have survived, the rattle likely just death throes.

Poor fellow. No one deserves that.

With a sigh of sadness, but also a bit of guilt-tinged relief, Bryan turned and headed on up the ascending path through the canyon. If he hurried, he could make the plateau before dark and set up camp.

True to the bobcat's word, he found the path even out as the sun clipped past the lip of the mountain range in the distance. He set up camp in an open area away from the rocks and any other resting rattlesnakes. After his long day of hard exertion, he slept soundly, for what felt like the first time since he left home.

Three days later, he located the towering stone to the left of the trail that marked a rest stop and watering hole the bobcat told him about. In the dimming light of the afternoon, he failed to notice the flickering light already emanating from the nook. Another rattle had his heart pounding in his chest. "I-I'm just looking for a place to camp and fill my canteen," he choked out, unsure of how close he was to danger.

A soft, slow hiss eased out like a sigh. "Come 'round. I ain't gonna bite ye. Just gave me a fright, ye did." The voice was monotone and crisp, but not hostile.

Bryan still stepped cautiously around the pillar and found, to his surprise, a fire roaring next to a small campsite. Curled up beside the blaze, a snake sat eyeing him.

"You're welcome to share my fire, buffalo, if you like."

"Um. Bison, actually. Common mistake." Bryan chuckled nervously. *You know better than this. Don't be rude.*

"Sorry if I scared ye. Been on edge lately."

"I know. I am well versed in many animal behaviors. Just surprised me, that's all."

"Aw, ye ain't gotta lie. I know what critters think 'bout my kind. Some of it's true. Most ain't. Name's Silas."

Bryan found his guard dropping quickly around the creature. Despite his naturally vicious appearance, the doctor could see that he was not tensed to strike, and in fact, had a certain laid-back quality about him. "Bryan. Pleasure to meet you."

The two spent the next hour sharing pleasantries and news of the road. Soon they were laughing and telling tales, the snake of his work as a tracker, and Bryan of his most ridiculous patient stories.

"All of his fur completely singed off. You'll never see anything like a bald bear," the doctor snorted. Silas chortled his wheezy chuckle along with him. Bryan paused, listening as the snake broke out into a cough at the end of the laughter.

"Here," Bryan said as he pulled a bundle of herbs from his backpack. "Mix a scoop of this with water twice a day. Should clear up that cough."

"Nah, I ain't worried."

"Truly. If you ignore it, it will develop into something serious."

"Well, you'd know best, wouldn't ye? I ain't never seen no doctor since I was a little noodle."

"Trust me. Take the medicine and check in with a doctor the next time you can."

"I'll be alright. Ain't no doctors round here. But you know, Bryan, I heard they buildin' a new hospital up through the pass. Hear they need people to help out. I'm sure they could use someone with yer skills."

"Really? That's great. Thank you for the tip."

"Thank you. I'd hate to wind up like my cousin. Got trapped under a rock. Couldn't get out. By the time we found him, he didn't last but a couple of days after. If only there had been someone around, someone we could have taken him to, or a place like that new hospital, he might've made it."

Bryan simply nodded as they bedded down across the fire from each other, the memory rising to choke him. Tears welled in his eyes at the thought of the poor snake, who he had seen and assumed to be a lost cause. If he hadn't been caught up in his fears and worries, he might have noticed the reptile was still alive.

A new determination stirred deep inside, fighting back against the dread that had been consuming him. Faint, but enough to give him a goal. A mission.

"That's' it," he whispered in the dark. "I'll find that hospital. A new place that really needs me. I'll start over."

Chapter Seven

Higher Calling

The Llama and the Bison

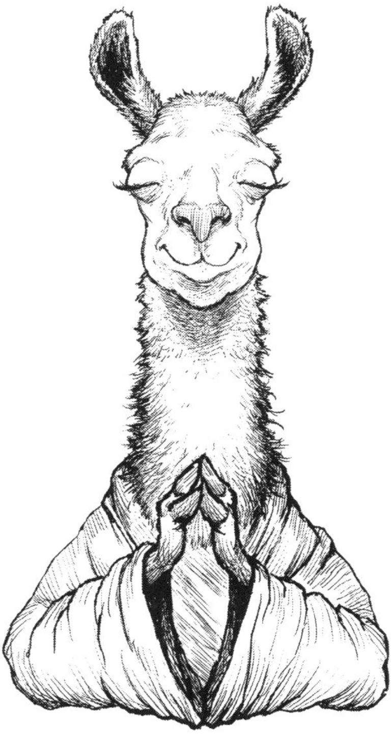

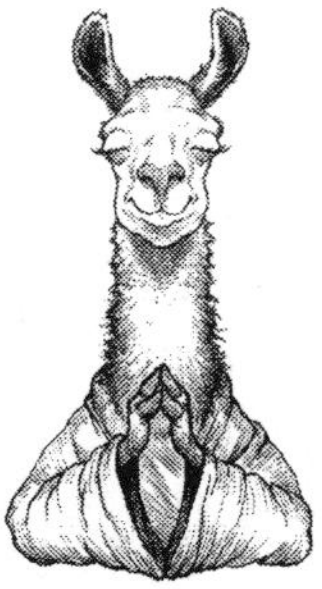

High in the mountains, the bison traveled the thin paths worn by rams' hoofs. The trek was difficult but rewarding in a way he had not encountered in years. After many hours, he came upon a lake, nestled in a hollow, lined with trees, picturesque and wholly peaceful.

There he sat down on a rock to eat and rest.

Before long, he fell asleep. When he awoke, he found he was not alone, for a llama grazed nearby, seemingly oblivious to his presence.

"Is this your valley, creature?" the bison asked.

At first, he wasn't sure if the strange creature heard him, but after chewing for a time, it said, "This valley is certainly mine, though I can claim no ownership. Rather, it has for a time claimed me. So too, it is yours, for now."

The llama's words sounded strange and circular to the bison's logical, linear mind.

"Then I can stay here for a time?"

"I am not sure," said the llama. "Can you?"

"I can help you and others; I am a healer. I will earn my place," the bison said earnestly.

"Who said you had to earn the right to be anywhere?"

Who gives us permission to live our lives?

ONE HOOF IN FRONT OF THE OTHER. Bryan had never climbed mountains before. Even heading up through the relatively open pass, increasing altitude made breathing a chore. Still, his resolve to reach his goal had not wavered. The rest of his confidence, however, was dulled by exhaustion and time. It took much longer to reach the mountains than he had hoped.

Days of having only himself to talk to, trapped in his thoughts, diluted some of the energy he had restored in finding a purpose. And again, he failed to see to the needs of others he passed. Mostly it was fatigue, bruises, blisters. Those would heal.

His final destination was more important than that, wasn't it? Once he reached the rumored location, he would be of better use to the area. Out here, he had to forage for medicinal herbs, create make-shift cures.

Of course, lying to oneself was harder to do the longer he did it. Spite fueled his decisions as much as any pragmatism or rationalizing.

If he wasn't allowed to help anyone without proper licensing, without approval from the animals in charge, then he wouldn't. In the back of his head, a voice tried to reason with his childish behavior, but he shoved it aside, buried it deeper.

The doctor reached a level area, pausing to catch his breath. The path ahead vanished into coniferous trees. Perhaps a rest and a bit of shade would help him clear his addled mind. He strolled on aching hoofs into the cluster of green needles and breathed deeply the sap and rich loamy soil.

"The worst patients in the world are doctors themselves," Professor Ermine lectured. "You'll know it when you push yourself too hard, when you do not rest in a crisis, endangering your patients' lives by neglecting your own needs. It is a difficult thing for anyone to take their own advice, for a doctor, even more so."

Wry laughter from a classroom full of would-be healers echoed in his memories. Dr. Ermine had been the one to inspire him to head back out west where he was from. To find a community in need and establish his practice.

"From time to time, diagnose yourself."

So, he did.

Aching hoofs and back. Muscle fatigue. Should stretch and massage the tissue, deeper, a twinge of sharp pain. Tendons. Cold and heat, alternating. Gentle, active recovery.

The mental exercise washed out a lot of the soured thought patterns he had indulged in throughout his sojourn. Soon he was smirking at his own assessment, lost in good memories of his early days of study—basic remedies, all but forgotten.

So distracted was he that he was knee deep in ice cold water before he realized he had cleared the trees and entered a broad, hollowed out basin. The lake swept out before him, impossibly blue, ringed by massive, vibrant green pines and firs. And beyond that, a ring of jagged, primordial rock thrust up into the crystal sky.

For several minutes, he simply stood there, letting the freezing water soothe his inflamed legs, reveling in the overwhelming peace of the place.

"I have never seen a bison swim before." A voice jolted him from his reverie.

Bryan turned and gaped at an animal he had only ever read about in books. The llama wore simple robes and small, round spectacles, standing casually on the shore and leaning on a cane of petrified wood.

"I was just doing some cold therapy. To reduce swelling." For some reason, he felt like a calf trying to excuse his actions to a mother cow.

"Wise, indeed. Much knowledge rests behind your eyes, friend." The llama smiled warmly. Calm radiated from the creature, soothing his embarrassment.

"Y-you're a llama. I have heard of animals like you." The doctor could not keep a tone of awe and wonder from his voice as he trudged slowly back to the pebbled beach. "Are you a holy man?"

"Holey? Yes. We all have holes inside, waiting to be filled. With possessions, with purpose, with love, with hate. We each choose what to fill ourselves with."

Bryan huffed a chuckle, not sure how to take the turn of phrase. He shook off some of the water soaking his lower half, sighing in relief as the strange animal gestured with his stick to follow him. It felt like an invitation, but also a gentle order.

It felt natural to fall in behind the llama as he turned and shuffled along, winding back up a broad path Bryan had not noticed. They walked in amicable silence for a time; the bison trying to decide what to ask first. Before he had a chance to utter a word, the elderly animal said, "You may call me Lham."

"Bryan Bison. It's very nice to meet you. May I ask where we are going?" He assumed there must be a lodging of some sort nearby where the creature lived. Lham said nothing for a time, and Bryan began to wonder if he heard him or was just ignoring his question. Just before them, the trees thinned, and the llama glanced back at him with a small smile on his face.

"We are going to where you are needed."

Bryan stepped through the brush and emerged onto a sweeping slope that ran down between two swells of the mountain and into a valley that curved off into the distance, farther than he could see. Rivers crisscrossed the fertile swells, and where the two largest met at the bottom of the slope, he saw an edifice, surrounded by a few smaller buildings.

"Is that the hospital? How did you know?"

"Because there is nothing else up here. Why else would a learned animal from the plains come to the mountains?" A mischievous smirk graced the llama's face as he teased the bison.

Bryan couldn't suppress a grin of his own. Of course. As they started down the slope, a million questions swarmed through his head.

He settled on a simple one: "Why build it here? Why not closer to a town, or city, where it's safer?"

"This is not a place without its dangers. But here, there is so much good to be done. There are fewer folk that need to reach us from the east, as you came and saw. However, in the west, there are many more animals, but things are far more primal."

The thought resonated within the doctor. Yes. This was exactly what he was looking for. This could be an adventure.

"The real question, however, is why you have come? To heal, or to be healed?"

The doctor started to answer but paused. He had the sinking suspicion that Lham already knew why he had come. That wasn't the real question either. Still, he could only answer simply, "I am a doctor. I would offer my skills at healing."

"Offer healing? Like a product you have for sale?"

"No, no. That's not what I meant."

His face must have betrayed his dismay because the llama reached out and rested a hand on his shoulder. "You wish to relieve the suffering of others."

"Yes."

A broad grin spread across the llama's wrinkled features. "And perhaps we will find a way to relieve yours as well."

Chapter Eight

The Definition of Pain

The Bison and the Cougar

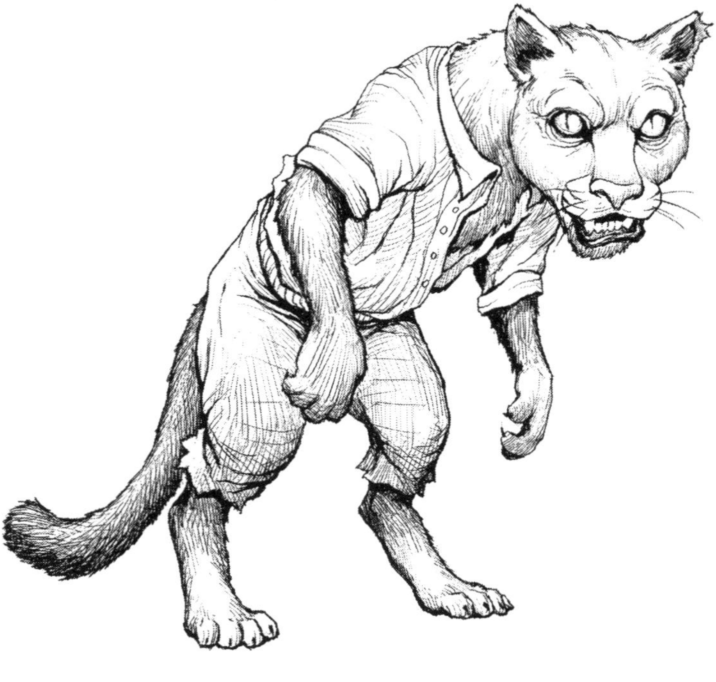

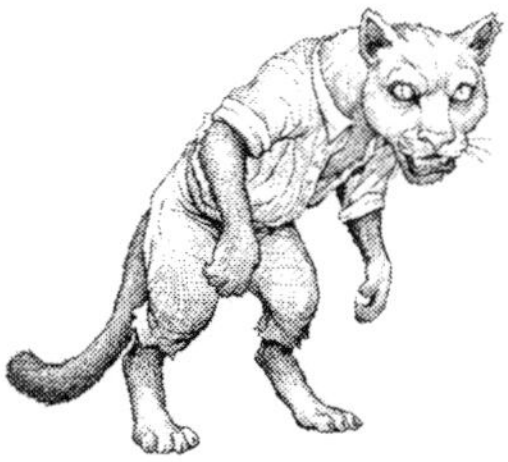

Months passed in the valley, and the bison found a new home for himself. Life was harder in the mountains, but with the combined effort of the animals who lived there, the small group of creatures thrived.

The llama knew many different animals who contributed to the greater good, the bison included, seeing to their health needs. After being driven from his previous home, having a purpose began to heal the bison's heart.

His new home was a haven. Safe.

However, one day as the bison was passing through a ravine on his way back from helping some of the high mountain animals, he heard a sound behind him. The hair on the back of his neck stood up. Instinct told him he was in danger.

As he slowly turned, he caught sight of a large cougar stalking him. He ran, but the starved predator was much faster and more agile than he was.

Realizing he could not flee to safety, the bison acted in desperation, leaping down the side of the ravine. But the cougar was just as desperate and leapt after him.

They tumbled to the bottom, stones and debris collapsing down the mountainside. When the dust settled, the sturdy bison had survived. The cougar did not.

Gravely injured, the bison despaired no one would find him and succumbed to unconsciousness. When he awoke, the bison found himself in the care of a dog. He had been rescued. But the pain in his back and leg were so overwhelming that the bison could not reason or think of anything else. Relief was the only thought in his mind, and he understood why creatures would do anything to make it go away.

Experiencing intense pain is the only way to truly understand how to treat pain.

DR. BISON BREATHED OUT THROUGH HIS NOSE into his face covering. Pulling a final stitch closed, he leaned back as Nurse Squirrel snipped the cord and proceeded to wrap the fresh suture.

The lean billy goat let out a tense breath as well and nodded his thanks to the doctor as he stood. “Let’s aim to not see you back in here for a bit, eh, Gill?” Bryan chuckled as he washed his hoofs in the basin.

“We-eh-eh-ell, Doc, can’t say as I can guarantee that. The mines are what they are.” The goat grinned at his statement, flashing several gold teeth. Gill had several new ones since his last visit.

Bryan shook his head, waving over his shoulder. He knew he didn’t even have to bother telling the old timer what to do with the wound.

The past year saw many folks like Gill become familiar faces, as well as the less frequent traveling sellers, hawkers, and herders who came through in season. And besides them, there was a steady and sometimes overwhelming stream of random creatures passing through. They needed odds and ends treated, rotten teeth pulled, and just about every type of injury and malady that could occur on the road and out in the sticks.

"Oh, before you go, doctor," Nurse Squirrel caught him just outside the door.

"Hmm?" he asked before it dawned on him what she was about to inquire about. Another sigh escaped his nostrils, this one a bit frustrated. The finicky nurse scrunched her face up apologetically. "Give him a two-week dose. I'll sign off on it."

Bobbing her head graciously, the fluffy tailed assistant zipped back in to deliver the good news to the constantly aching worker. The stitches were usually the most serious of the goat's injuries, but he sported bruises, sprains—the life of a miner was rough work.

Lost in thought, Doctor Bison nearly bowled into a slender, furry fellow coming around the corner. Lham casually sidestepped, avoiding from bumping into the bison.

"Good afternoon, my friend."

"Lham, how are you?" They fell into step as Bryan continued down the hallway.

"I am."

The bison nearly rolled his eyes at the telling response. He had become quite fond of the elder llama over the past year and the animal's affectations and pleasant nature. There was always a sense of calm and peace radiating in Lham's vicinity.

"Was there something I could help you with?"

"Ah, yes. I was to fetch you to see Doctor Labrador. He needed a second opinion."

Allowing Lham to lead the way, the two proceeded into another examination room where an alert, energetic dog, Doctor Louis Labrador, was looking through a microscope at a sample. Just through another door, a fox sat patiently on the table, waiting for the doctor to return.

"Bryan, glad he found you. This fox appears to have some sort of anemia, or possibly dehydration. I can't tell by the initial sample we took."

Nodding, Doctor Bison moved to the stool to look for himself. "Hmm. Well, it may be a matter of volume, Louis. Let's get a full blood sample, urine, and stool and we can run a series of tests? If the symptoms are conflicting or obscure, we should be able to ascertain a more definitive diagnosis in a day or two. He isn't in dire straits, is he?"

"No, no. Finn, would you come here for a moment?" Doctor Labrador called.

The fox in question rose and leaned into the room looking anxious. "Yessir?"

His face was sallow, his fur a bit matted and greasy. Bryan noted the glassy look in his eyes, the dry nose. After a moment of looking the fox over, checking his ears, throat and checking the file for his temperature, he clapped the fox on the back. "Don't worry too much, Finn. I would wager you've got a secondary infection. You have a fever or cold recently?"

"Hmm. Sure did."

"I thought as much. All the same, we will take some samples before we run a few tests to be sure." Bryan paused, looking back over his shoulder and winking, "Louis should have your *lab* work back in a day or two."

A second passed, the four creatures froze. All at once everyone but Doctor Labrador burst out laughing. Lham's chortle, in particular, rang out like bells through the hall. The dog rolled his eyes, shaking his head, eventually succumbing to a chuckle.

* * *

The days passed in a similar fashion, making rounds, visiting nearby homes on call, and helping with the daily upkeep around the hospital facility. More than anything, what stood out to the wayward doctor was that he was actually *helping* those in need, doing the duty that he had sworn himself to. For the first time in a long while, Bryan felt he was truly changing people's lives for the better.

This residency at the hospital in the mountains lifted a weight off his shoulders. Even with the pressure of being one of two doctors in a relatively busy area, the energy of the craft and the new challenges it presented every day kept Bryan driven and passionate. And it helped to ease the guilt of having left his community behind, leaving them to the fate of that horrid system. What else could he have done, though?

Here, he was respected. Needed.

The only drawback to the workload was the lack of rest. But the turnabout was that he constantly felt refueled by his original desire to go into medicine. There was the look of hope from the gopher, who thought he wouldn't dig again, the smile of relief from the mother rabbit, the runt of her litter safely delivered. Every creature had an inherent need for care, but none so much as these animals out in the wilderness. And at a hospital where they did not ask for much in payment, the small and scattered community provided what they could in thanks, giving to each other in effort and time and resources for the betterment of the whole.

Otherwise, the hospital survived on donations from unlikely and often surprising beneficiaries. Several wealthy caravans of merchants gave gifts of materials and money as they passed through to ensure all travelers would have access to help. D.L. Lham seemed to have other connections, ensuring that they generally received everything they needed to continue.

Unfortunately, not all their provisions were guaranteed. They had not received a shipment of pain-relieving medicine in some time.

"Seriously, Bryan?" Doctor Labrador slapped the folder down on Bison's desk.

Dr. B didn't bother to look up from his notes, knowing exactly what it was about. He also did not want to see the look on the black-furred face. "What's the difference, Lou? Who are we saving it for?"

"Serious emergencies."

"Is any patient's pain less of an emergency than another?"

"Yes. We have to make that call. I know you're compassionate, but your bleeding heart is putting us in a bind. Gill Goat will be in pain no matter what. You could have told him he needs to wait or purchase other remedies from a caravan."

Bryan sighed. "Maybe you're right. I'll ease up on handing out prescriptions."

"Thank you, Bryan." Doctor Lab nodded, tapping the door frame as he left the room.

But the issue was far from over in Bryan's mind, his thoughts lingering on the topic for days after.

What gives us the right to tell anyone their pain isn't as valid as others?

* * *

The return trip from the alpine meadows always felt longer than the journey out. Several families of pikas, marmots, and birds lived in the rocky terrain above the tree line, and once a month, Bryan or Louis made the trek to set up a station they could all come to and receive vaccines and other needs.

He had just entered the tree line, pausing for a water break, when he felt a shiver run up his spine. Bryan looked around, his eyes darting back and forth in the dimming dusk light. The fur standing up on the nape of his neck told him something was trailing him. He felt the stabbing claws of terror scrape across his skin, sinking down into his hoofs. *You shouldn't have stayed so late.*

But he had made the trip dozens of times now. He never encountered a predator before. His instincts, however, didn't lie.

Slinging his canteen onto his shoulder, Bryan slowly eased up to his hoofs. The path might offer a little more safety, being relatively well traveled. He made it down and around a bend on the slope, hoping to make it up and over the rise where he would be within sight of the small town and hospital.

A low growl and a light shuffle told him it was too late.

Logically, he knew he shouldn't run, shouldn't make himself into prey. Something deep inside of the doctor took over, a primal mind that only knew that he had to get away, had to run, escape whatever was stalking him. He took off abruptly at a full gallop. A good ways back behind him, he heard a scrape and scrabble of claws on rock.

A snarl in the brush, back in the trees to his left.

Frantically, Bryan tried to think of anything he could do to deter his assailant and distract them. His breath came in labored gasps, panic threatening to choke him. *Think. Don't let fear blind you.*

Somewhere in his mind, a plot formed. There was a small alcove along the path just ahead. He rushed to the right as he came around a scree of rock, and he threw himself against the wall, his chest heaving as he tried to stay quiet. The sun was almost gone, but he had just enough light to see the cougar ease out of the trees, its green eyes gleaming in the near dark.

Those eyes held no anger or rage to complement his terror and desperation. Only hunger resided. Bryan forced calm into his voice, clinging with every ounce of his will to remain still.

"Please. You don't have to do this. We have food. We have water," he spoke softly but steadily, much steadier than he felt. "We have anything you could need down at the hospital. If you'll just come with me. I'm a doctor."

This creature was beyond words. Starvation had clearly drawn its skin up inside its ribs. Reasoning would do no good. So, Bryan waited for the right moment to enact his hasty plan.

Just before the creature could lower itself into a crouch to pounce, the bison reached back and grabbed the lowest bough of the tree behind him, yanking with all of his substantial strength.

The roots of the tree wound through the cliffside, tangled in the dirt and stone. As he pulled, a resounding crack echoed out through the hills, just before a tumble and clatter of rock.

Bryan shouted out as he dove to the side, trying to escape the fall. The cougar was not so lucky, however. Boulders as big as his head, some as big as his entire body, rained down, crashing into the narrow gap.

And all Bryan could do was cover his head with his hoofs and pray. An explosion of pain followed, in his back and leg, and the bison blacked out.

Chapter Nine

Alternative Lifestyles

The Bison and the Opossum

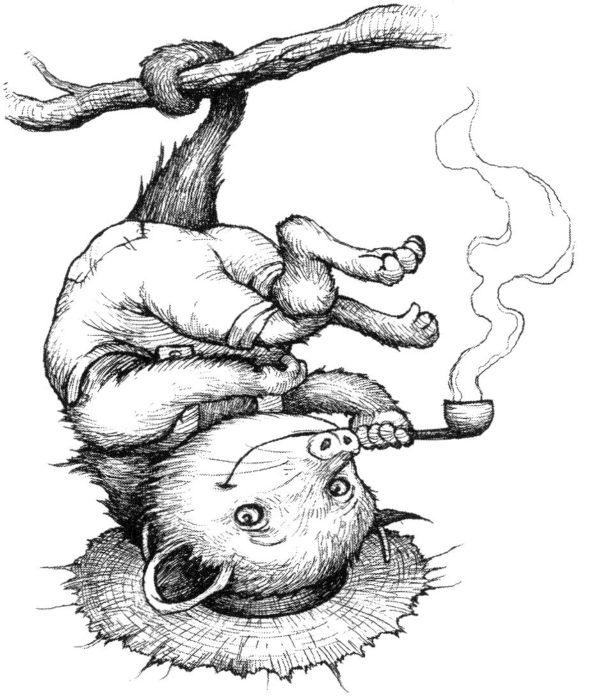

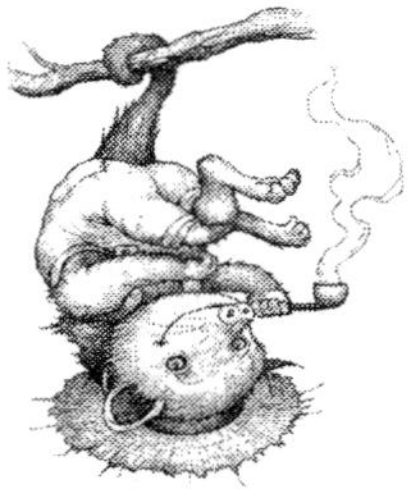

The bison had many patients, but he had rarely been one himself, not since he was very young. He had sustained broken bones, a cracked hoof, a chipped tooth, when he was a young bison. Since then, the memories of that sort of pain had fallen far into the background. But now, in his newfound injuries, he realized the extent of the suffering that his own patients went through.

Objectively, he always believed he could relate, but living it was altogether different.

"I cannot bear this pain," the bison cried. He knew he needed to manage it in order to heal.

So, the dog helped as best he could, administering what medicines he had. Yet nothing seemed to work.

One day, the llama came to the bison and said, "If you are willing to try, there might be something that could help you with your pain."

"I'll do anything," the bison pleaded.

Thus, the llama sought out the opossum and brought him to the bison. Now, the dog was skeptical of the treatments the opossum offered, counseling the bison to refuse, to stay true to the accepted methods of healing.

Pain won out, and he immediately noticed the results. As his pain subsided, he thought to himself, what other treatments have I ignored or dismissed because I was too close-minded?

Desperation tests conviction. Pain shakes resolve. Relief can change the way a creature thinks.

* * *

FEVERISH DREAMS DROVE BRYAN back to a soaked, thrashing consciousness.

He sat up, instantly regretting the jerking movement as his back screamed in protest.

A few weeks had crawled by since the incident of the rockslide, the rescue team, and the emergency surgery Doctor Labrador performed to stop the bleeding and set the bone in his leg. Each day Bryan agonized, writhing in bed when he wasn't in a fitful sleep, exhausted from hours of trying to lie still.

The medicine kept the worst of it at bay the first week. Now, the additional angst and physical withdrawal from the opiates added another layer of discomfort.

"Hey, what are you doing up?" Louis happened by the door, looking up from a chart.

"Ugh. I have to move around." The bison gingerly eased himself over the edge of the bed. "I just can't take this. Lying around. Bored out of my mind. Need a distraction from the pain."

Doctor Labrador hustled to his side as he tried to stand, firmly pressing him back down to sit. "Whoa, there. You need bed rest. I know it's trying, but you could seriously hurt yourself again if you fell."

"I need to do something, Lou. This is intolerable. Don't we have anything left for the pain?"

A sad shake of his head, ears flopping gently. "Still no word.

Lham sent word and another order. We're hoping for something by the end of the month, but that's being overly optimistic, in my opinion. There's been a shortage. You know that as well as I do." The implication of their previous arguments was heavy in his tone.

"You're right. Besides, we have patients that need care a lot more than I do, with what little medicine we have left."

"That tiny stockpile is also my fall back if we get any busier with the monsoon season starting. We've got our paws full without you to help at the moment."

"Which is another reason I need to get up and about. There must be some way I can still help. Rolling bandages—anything."

Louis paused in the doorway, shaking his head with a soft chuckle. "You really are resilient as a mush dog, Doc. I'll see if we can have you assist Nurse Squirrel with some unguents and topicals tomorrow, okay?"

Bryan slumped back, suddenly feeling exhausted. *Tomorrow, then.*

* * *

"You're going to wear a trench in the floorboards. Should we hitch a plow to you instead?"

Bryan grimaced, turning to greet the elder llama standing in the doorway of his office. He was spending more time at his desk, more often standing and pacing rather than sitting. Louis sat at his desk through the adjoining door, studying a new manual they received the previous week on insect stings and bites. Ticks had been a huge problem over the summer.

The Doctor paused in his hobbling, leaning against his desk. "Honestly, I'd welcome the work. I'm still too weak and shaky to do much more than quick examinations and paperwork."

“It takes time, my friend.” Lham’s pleasant, singsong voice clashed with the irritation the words affected in the bison.

“That’s what everyone keeps saying. I can self-diagnose.”

“Yet you won’t take your own advice.” Louis grumbled from the next room. Before Bryan could make a snide response, Lham interjected.

“I think you need a distraction. I know of a farm not too far from here. I need you to fetch a package from the owner for me. And perhaps you may discover some relief of a different nature in the process,” Lham chimed, smiling slightly.

Doctor Labrador, overhearing from his desk, frowned and shook his head. “The walk would do you good, sure. But be wary of anything *that* farmer tries to give you.”

Bryan cocked an eyebrow. Louis was rather conservative in his practice, but what could this be that had the dog’s hackles rising?

A short time later, Lham helped Bryan in winding the back brace tightly around him and waited while he adjusted his crutch and situated his shoulder bag. The pair slowly made their way to the hospital’s side entrance.

“So, what’s this package I’m picking up? And what’s this other business that has the Lab in a tizzy?”

“Tea, for me. For you, let this be a consideration for alternative methods of treatment. Keep an open mind. It’s best for you to see for yourself, and to decide what you think, without bias. Head north and east of town.” Lham waved as he shuffled onto the path. It was perhaps the most direct the llama had ever been with him.

Bryan took his time wandering out of the cluster of buildings that made up what could arguably be called a town around the hospital. The exercise was invigorating, but he knew better than to overdo it, especially knowing he had to get all the way to the farm and back. He had a vague idea of where the homestead was, having traveled this path before to see several nearby families in the hills.

The trek out to the farm took a lot more out of him than he hoped. His arm ached from leaning on his crutch and his joints were stiff from more activity that he had done in months. Seeing the low fence and gate gave him a bit of energy and relief that he could take a much-needed break before heading back. A cottage sat a way back from the worn, wooden slatted gate, fields stretching off into the distance over the hill behind the quaint structure. As he made his way onto the path inside the gate, he tried to make out what sort of plant was growing, acre upon acre, under canvas canopies in the fields beyond. It reminded him of something he couldn't quite put his finger on. His initial thought had been poppies, based on Louis's reaction, but the color was wrong. And why the tarps?

No one stepped out to greet him, and he was about to knock on the door, when he noticed something odd around the side of the house, under the hanging laundry on the lines. Heading around the corner, he squinted as the billowing sheets moved again and he caught sight of a tail?

A tremor shook Bryan as he hustled as quickly as he could manage, pulling aside the sheet. Below him, a possum lay on the ground, its tongue hanging out, its feet in the air.

"Oh my goodness, you poor thing," he muttered as he tried to crouch down to check for a pulse. As he did so, the possum sprang back to life, startling him enough to send him sprawling back on his bottom.

"Goodness," he shouted, feeling embarrassed that he fell for the age-old trick.

"Oh sorry, there friend," the small, rather ugly creature crooned. "I thought you were a predator, or someone come to take my plants.

Or worse."

Its tone and voice belied any worry over such things, like he was as relaxed as he could possibly be. Bryan almost started laughing outright at the ridiculous animal as he adjusted his overalls and straw hat. He should have known.

Taking the bison's flustered reaction in stride, the old critter turns on its paw and headed toward the back porch. "Old family trick, you know? I guess rather I should say it's an old trick of the species."

"Oh, I am very familiar," Bryan chuckled, rising awkwardly to follow. "I'm a physician over at the hospital down in town."

"Ah, yes. Yes, I've heard of you. Dr. Bison, isn't it?"

"Yes, that's me. Albeit a little worse for wear right now."

"Looks like you didn't take your own care too serious, eh?" The possum produced a little wooden pipe and gestured to the crutch, smiling ruefully. "Well, from what I hear, wasn't your fault that you wound up in this predicament. Dangerous, them mountains is."

A peaceful air hung around the cozy patio and the owner of the land. Bryan sighed as he settled himself on the large tree stump across from the tiny rocking chair the possum eased back into. "That is more or less why I'm here. Mister . . ."

"You can call me Ogle, Ogle Opossum. Yes, sir. Family name, you see." He winked as he finished. "I've got Lham's packet ready inside, but that's not what you were gettin' at, was it?"

Ogle lit the little pipe with a stick from an oil lantern by the door. A cloying, pungent aroma filled the air.

Ah, so that is what is growing in the fields.

Bryan pondered for a moment. He knew exactly what the possum was smoking. But he wasn't keen on getting intoxicated. On the other hoof, he knew the plant had pain relieving capabilities when smoked. Still, he had never tried the drug himself.

May as well ask. Lham wouldn't send me here for no reason.

"We're waiting on a shipment of medicines to come in from town. It's well overdue. Bandits intercepted one already. Since then, there have been shortages, weather—long story. We have nothing to help me manage my pain." *And the suffering I have gone through from coming off the medication.*

"Ah, yes. I have heard. Hindered me and my kin a bit, too, gettin' a few things we need out here. However, you see, I am real careful about who I give what to, if you catch my meaning? My primary crop is made predominantly for cloth, rope, paper. My plants are a very diverse crop. We can use them for a world of products and services. Least of which being well, what you're here for."

"I don't mean to impose. Lham simply suggested that I collect his package for him and inquire about any assistance you might offer. And honestly, I don't want to get—"

"Higher than a kite at the country fair?" The possum grinned. "Ain't the only thing we can do."

Bryan was at a loss for words, laughing along with the kindly creature. He waited patiently, not knowing where this was going.

"Now, if Lham trusts you, and you'll trust me through him, we have some other products. Nothing I would recommend going straight into surgery after using, it. But they can help you get back to where you need to be."

"That would be incredible. My issue was that I do not want to be incapacitated. I need to at least help around the hospital until I am back at one hundred percent. Otherwise, I could easily drink my hurt away."

"Hmm. It's a bit of a far stretch of comparison between the two, but I see where you're comin' from. Can't perform the complicated stuff while influenced."

"Precisely. And I don't plan to do so while taking any sort of opiate. I just need to sleep, to sit still and get paperwork done, for now."

"Well, I think I might have something that will help, regardless. See, my wife and I make oil from the plant as well. It's an extract if you will, and it doesn't have the same effects as the more *recreational* aspects of the plant, if you will. Might do you some good, though, a puff or two to loosen up and relax."

"Really?" The doctor was intrigued.

He heard the plant had many uses, but the only one most common folk knew of was smoking it. Several local young coyotes used to smoke out by the creek when he was just a calf, laughing hysterically as they coughed up a storm.

After a moment of deliberation, Bryan shrugged. What harm could come from trying it? He didn't have any responsibilities in the near future that it could compromise. Sensing his shift in mood, Ogle smiled and offered him a puff.

"Why don't you come inside for some tea, and I'll see what I can find for you." Ogle stood, waving the coughing bison along.

A bison whose back pain was already subsiding.

Chapter Ten

Pursuing Happiness

The Bison and the Cow

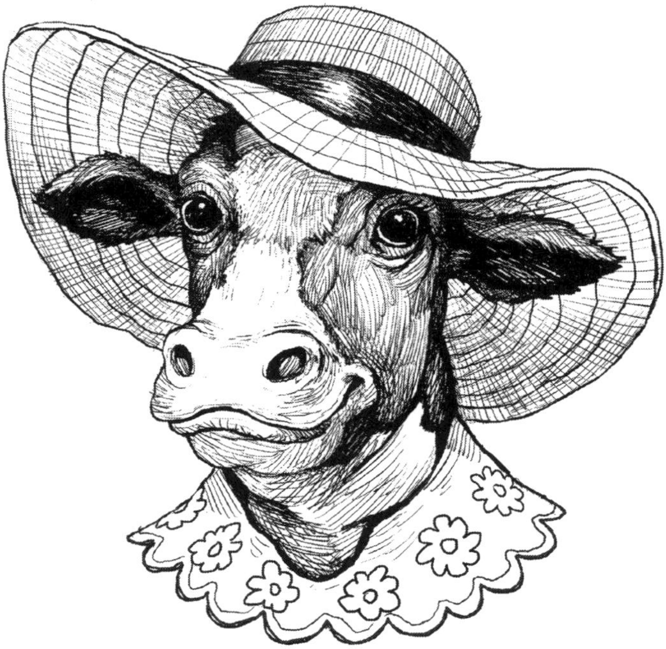

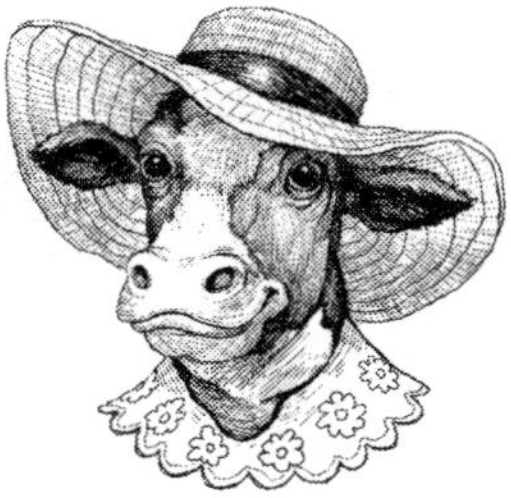

During his years in the wilderness, the bison found a place to serve in his duties as a healer, and he was opening up and learning who he wanted to be. Nonetheless, as he healed from his physical injuries, and challenged himself mentally, he realized one aspect of his being was lacking: friendships.

The bison often felt lonely, longing for companionship, not just peers of like-mind, but of like-heart and spirit, as well. He cared deeply for all the other animals, but he did not know how to let them provide care for him.

Being a healer, he had always done the healing.

One day, as the bison was dipping in a lake, seeking relief from the heat, he came upon a very pleasant looking cow, chewing cud nearby. Nothing about the creature doing what cows do seemed out of place, but the way she seemed to truly enjoy what she was doing took him off guard. He longed for that kind of peace.

As he came to know the cow, he realized she was unlike anyone he had ever met. They shared many of the same interests, and she was incredibly intelligent. Yet she was much more relaxed about all of it than he was.

At first, he thought this might be a lack of ambition. Soon he understood how wrong he was. On a long walk one afternoon, he asked about this, how she could balance work and recreation.

The cow smiled and said, "There's more to living than just success at work or health of mind and body. One must also foster relationships with others on an equal footing."

"I have peers," he said.

"Not peers, but close friends. Those with whom you might share your creativity, your hobbies, your interests outside of the practice of your work."

The Bison realized he wanted these things but did not know how to find them.

Health is about learning to thrive, not just survive.

BRYAN SIGHED, TILTING BACK HIS HEAD and blocking the blaring sun from his eyes with one hoof. Reaching down, he scooped a ladle of cool water from the bucket beside him and took a long draw before dumping the rest on his head.

"Working yerself into a lather again, I see, Doc?" Eugenia Ewe bleated as she trotted by on the way to her flower garden.

"I may need to stop by for a new cake of soap when I finish." Bryan called after her, eliciting a throaty cackle. The goats' scents and soaps were one of a kind, and they had even developed an herbal, antibacterial version for use at the hospital with the help of the crafty lady.

Bryan stretched his back, the occasional stiff twinge finding its way into the muscles. After another ladle of water, the big bison got back to work, pulling weeds, ignoring the heat.

The sun in the mountains was more intense, but most days, wind and cooler temperatures balanced it to a tolerable level. Today was not one of those days, but luckily, the water he splashed himself with caught the sparse breeze and offered some relief.

Regardless of the higher temperatures, Doctor Bison was enjoying hard labor, spending time outdoors and doing physical activity again. The small mountain community was growing around the hospital, and with it, the need for sustainability. Thus, the members of the burgeoning town started a garden of crops in the west field. While everyone contributed, Bryan found himself a task-oriented activity that quickly returned him to his former fitness and more. He worked in the garden at least every other day, between patients and in his downtime.

Long walks and even runs became a staple of his routine. His leg might as well never been broken.

Several months slipped by in this way, and he was truly feeling a sense of peace. The injuries that incapacitated him resulted in a very different outcome to what he ever could have expected.

First, he was forced to stop working constantly, something he threw himself into the first year he was at the mountain hospital. Months of insufficient rest wore him down emotionally and mentally.

Second, by getting back to the outlying homes and through his connection with Lham and the Opossum family, he spent a much larger portion of his time with the other animals in the valley system. He found like-minded peers and even made some very close friends. Prior to fleeing, he never got closer to anyone other than work colleagues or patients. And instead of the worry that he would falter or become compromised in his medical integrity and fortitude, he felt more whole as a creature than ever before.

It also had a lot to do with creating the place he lived in for himself and claiming it as his own. The garden, the expansion to the hospital's recovery wing, and the new operating theater all took shape with his direct input and oversight, and he was even fairly vocal as a leading member of the community council.

While the days often seemed to fly by, he somehow found more time for the things he loved. Shipments finally resumed, both on the medicinal side of things, as well as trade and provisional caravans. This meant there was far more access to books, art, and music from the traveling bands who paid for their stay and treatment in town by performing for the locals.

The steady influx of animals had another benefit—diversity. Personally, the two doctors benefited from a few new doctors and nurses who spent weeks or months at the hospital to learn new skills from Doctor Bison and Doctor Labrador, furthering the capacity of the hospital and helping to spread the knowledgeable base of medical practitioners in the lands out west. They became the premiere station for frontier medicine, and every town, village, and tribe wanted their healers to learn from the intrepid doctors. And just as his professors in medical school had often recounted, teaching shifted his perspective on his craft. It forced him to find new ways to relay the methods that led to new ideas and a diligence for service he hadn't previously felt.

Interactions with patients were far more meaningful. He gleaned lessons from each patient and started documenting every encounter with great care. He maintained a journal where he recorded both his experiences and the medical findings.

Doctor Labrador was also thriving. His collection of textbooks grew, and he was publishing unusual cases in his own medical journal. All the attention was even helping to curb his restless tendencies.

They learned so much in such a short time, and their friendship finally overcame their differences as they taught together. They challenged each other and helped creatures they both cared for.

Bryan smiled as he noticed Louis out beside the building on the shady grounds, napping contentedly. After gathering up his tools and depositing them back in the shed, he headed into town to see about getting some soap for a much-needed bath.

Strange smells and a bustle about the little town caught his attention as he strolled down the only street between the dozen or so buildings. There appeared to be an impromptu pop-up market at the far end of the street, not uncommon, with so many more traveling merchants these days.

"What's all the fuss about, Jimmy?" Doctor B waved as one of the Marmot's boys walked by, clearly on an errand.

"Oh, some group o' medicine women set up shop selling herbs and natural rem'dies, Doc. Ma's all a tizzy over the honeycomb. This's my third trip out to pick stuff up she done bought." The serious little fellow shook his head, rolling his eyes at his mother.

"Thanks for the info. Good luck, Gary."

"Harumph. Yer welcome, Doc B," Gary nodded, grumbling his woes as he scuffled along.

The bison greeted a few more locals on his way to the canvas-topped cluster. Most of the stalls were simple—clusters of roots, stems, flowers. The usual fare of peddled pickings from the countryside. One booth, true to the gopher's word, was buzzing with little bees, a wagon parked at the back full of what appeared to be a mobile beehive.

"Wonders never cease. You ever seen anything like it?" A smooth, laughter-filled voice reached Bryan from the side of the last building in town, a newer construction he had been meaning to check out.

Along the side of the house, a cluttered, fenced-in area shaded in colorful tarps exploded with color and smell. Flowers he had never seen, scents of herbs he thought he recognized, all mingled together in a fragrant assault on the senses.

Then it clicked; it reminded him very distinctly of Mister Owl's apothecary.

But instead of dark, mysterious, and dusty, the whole place was vibrant, fresh, and cozy in a summer-day kind of way. He could tell it was very much the same in function. And there, sitting on a fairly new looking rocking chair among the blossoms, was a prettily dressed cow in a bright yellow dress and a matching sun hat to boot. She was weaving together several stalks of some plant, making a bracelet or a necklace.

Realizing the comment had been aimed at him, Bryan realized he was gawking a bit and cleared his throat. "Oh, truly. I didn't even know you could move a hive. Though I don't know much about bees, to be honest, except how to treat stings and such."

You're blathering.

The cow nodded, smiling at his flustered response. "You're the famous Doctor Bison, then?"

"Why yes, that would be me," he admitted, realizing the question was rhetorical. He chuckled a bit, stepping over to offer his hoof in greeting. "Doctor Bison. But you can call me Bryan."

"Cora Cow. It's very nice to put a face to the name everyone is always chattering about."

"I'd imagine you can't have heard much, being new in town." Bryan knew she couldn't have been here long if he had not met her yet. He knew everyone in town. Well, everyone knew everyone in town. Nonetheless, he had been out afield a bit the past few weeks making rounds.

"Oh, you'd be surprised. Not too many folks here that don't mention you in just about any and every conversation."

"Guess that comes with the territory."

"Somehow I think there's a bit more to it than that, but I appreciate the humility." She winked as she hid a smile.

"It was very nice to meet you, Miss Cora, but I really need to get down to the lake for a bath." Bryan felt his face heat up as his voice dropped off. He smirked as the cow raised an eyebrow.

Way to overshare, Bryan.

"Oh, please do. You smell terrible."

Bryan cocked his head back as a burst of laughter exploded out of him. All he could manage as a goodbye was a wave over his shoulder as he headed back toward Eugenia's.

"I hope we run into one another soon, Cora," he said, more to himself than out loud.

And they did.

A few days later, Bryan was out walking near the pond when Cora swept up alongside him, as if they had been walking together all along. He glanced at her, smiling a bit incredulously, and she returned his grin. "You know, you really ought to relax a bit more."

"What would call this, right now?"

"Oh, it's certainly a break from your work. But it's just that. You are always working, even when you are not at the hospital. And I would be very surprised if you weren't thinking about either the crops, the upcoming town hall meeting, or one, if not all, of your patients."

"Huh. Seems like you have me figured out. But I enjoy my job. And my other activities, challenging though they may be."

"Hmm."

"Besides all of that, I spend a very reasonable portion of my time reading, even for fun."

"I will give you that. However, from what I hear, you never go for a swim, other than to bathe, you never nap out on the green like your fellow Louis, and you rarely, if ever, attend gatherings in town that are not related to making the place run."

Bryan felt the incredulous look spreading over his face again and schooled it back to neutral. Cora was quite presumptuous, but he was charmed. She was not only observant, but intuitive. Still, he couldn't for the life of him decide why.

"If you don't mind me asking, why do you care?"

Cora looked at him like he spat in her soup. "Do I need a reason? To care about anyone? Especially someone who seems to be rather irreplaceable to this town."

"I'm not convinced." He was being a little difficult on purpose, and she raised an eyebrow to show she saw right through it. "Why go to all that trouble to find out about me?"

"*Maybe* I happen to want to be your friend. You're not from this area at all, much like myself. You're traveled and well read. Not to slight anyone from the area. It's just—"

"Sometimes you need to relate to someone."

"Ah, he's not completely oblivious," she laughed.

"Yet why do I feel like there's more to it?"

Cora slowed, a small frown furrowing her cream-colored brow. "Always diagnosing, hmm? Fine." They continued walking, entering a small grove of peach trees as she gathered her thoughts. "Apothecaries must understand the fundamentals of the compounds and base elements they use to make medicines. In my opinion, this must come not only from studying and rote memorization, but from a keen and natural intuition for the nature of things, a talent to be built on. And an ability to expand on for those who aren't so inclined."

"I'm following your lecture so far," Bryan smirked.

"I know, I tend to wax away poetically. What I mean is, to understand the whole, you must understand the parts. And be able to see when something is missing."

"And you think I'm missing something?"

"I do. I have seen it many times. I have lived through it in my own life."

"I feel more fulfilled than I ever have in my practice, my calling. I have real friends here. And a purpose outside my job, as well. So where am I lacking?" His question was genuine, earnest.

Cora turned to face him, smiling her small, knowing smile. "You do not *lack*, Bryan. You simply need to open up your spirit to express itself. You are a doctor. You are a leader. But those are *things* you are, that you do. Not *who* you are, not how others see you."

Bryan tried and failed to wrap his mind around the idea. He tended to think objectively, and clearly this was a very subjective conversation. A sigh hissed through his teeth as he thought of what to say. "Honestly, I have been feeling that way. Lham has all but said exactly the same since I arrived. But I don't know how to go there."

"Well, sometimes you just need a *guide*."

Chapter Eleven

Secret Calling

The Bison and the Elk

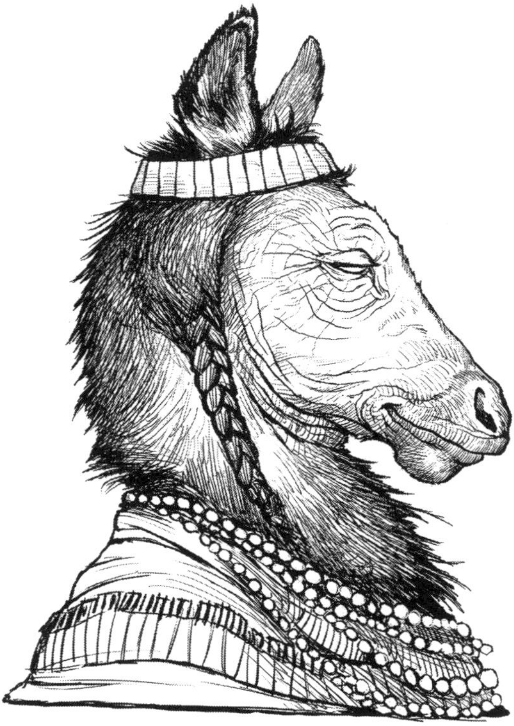

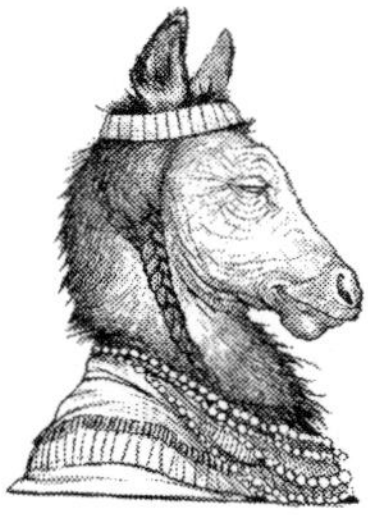

Throughout the years wandering afield, the bison encountered creatures of every shape and size, custom and instinct. They all had a unique influence on his healing, showing him great revelations in how to properly care for all animals.

It wasn't until he came upon a herd of elk high in the mountains, however, that he discovered something about himself. The herd invited him in, and he realized he had never seen such a large group of one animal any place, let alone a group that worked together for the benefit of the entire herd.

He stayed with them for a time and learned many things. Intriguingly, the elk cows oversaw the herd with little interference from the bulls. And with that came a different sort of leadership, one that he had never seen before.

At the end of his days with the elk learning the ways of the mothers, the elk matron asked him, "What is your purpose for healing? What is your purpose in life?"

For the first time, the bison was able to say, "I am a healer, but I'm also someone who needs to be healed."

And with that admission, the bison's heart opened to new possibilities.

Discovering the truth leads to professing the truth, which leads to action.

THE BURLY BISON BREATHED DEEPLY of the high mountain air. He felt tired from his hike, but in the best way possible. As he crested a moss-coated rise, highland grasses gently rustled to the ever-shifting winds. He gasped, his breath swept away by the sprawl of the valley below him, the verdant mountains sweeping out to the horizon.

Unbelievable.

In the two years he spent here, he could never get over the stunning landscape. His home and heritage would always be the plains, the rolling grass, but the primitive and primal nature of his new home had brought out a side of him he would never wish to live without. Here, at times, he had to be rugged, tough. A fine contrast to his compassionate medical practice and the warmth of the friendships he had developed at the hospital.

Still, he felt like something was missing, a third point in a triangle that he couldn't quite figure out. The sensation started growing as he got more and more comfortable with himself and his role as a leader and a healer. It doubled as he spent time with Cora, becoming fast friends with the herbalist. She was challenging in spiritual ways, asking all the right questions and more often than not, prodding him along to answers he intuitively wanted to know about himself.

She was also humorous to a fault, keeping him constantly in stitches. He couldn't remember any time in his life that he laughed so much as he had in the past few weeks.

Bryan smiled, shouldering his pack once more. As he trudged down the rocky descent, eager to reach his destination, he felt that certain something again, drawing him on. Pulling him.

Maybe it's just my curiosity about my upcoming patients.

Lham received a notice a week back from a local tribe of elk who needed a medicine man to come and assist them with some instruction, as well as bringing a case of needed materials. Bryan's large pack contained antiseptics, antibiotics, and a whole trove of other useful tools. He also planned to instruct them on how to use many of the ingredients they already had access to in new and innovative ways.

What captivated him most about this trip was that the tribe was notoriously insular. From all the accounts Dr. Bison found, they also had a reputation for being hardy creatures with an astoundingly low death rate.

Bryan reached the base of the incline, making his way around the large, serene lake that dominated the bowl-like enclosure that started the tribe's traditional grounds. As he rounded a slog of marshy clover and muck, he spotted a young elk bull waiting for him on a rock ahead.

The eager young buck perked up, noticing the doctor, and waved enthusiastically as he trotted to meet him.

"Doctor, Doctor, it's just so good to see you." His eyes lit up as he spoke, nearly bursting with excitement. "I am Moss of the Stoneherd. I have earned the privilege to meet you in person. I am the strongest of our young warriors."

"It is a pleasure to meet you, young warrior, and I'm honored by your escort." Dr. Bison smiled warmly and bowed just slightly. The elk's eyes widened at the gesture, on the verge of offense. Or embarrassment?

Clearly, the doctor would need to be careful handing out what appeared to be excessive compliments if he were to fit in. Or outright insulting the heads of this tribe, which would be far worse.

He gestured for the young buck to lead them on.

The two wandered along in amicable silence for quite a while before Moss spoke up again. Bryan could tell the youth was teaming with questions but was doing his best not to lose face or honor.

"It is unusual for them. To ask for an outsider to come."

Bryan thought about it for a time, how best to respond. He nodded to show that he had heard and was thinking. "I believe your elders are wise in both respects. For maintaining their autonomy, having the forethought to stay in touch with someone such as Lham, who would never interfere unless asked, and for seeking assistance when there might be no other solution." The implications of the statement by the elk told the doctor a few things about how their tribe worked. It also raised several questions. He had the feeling he wasn't just being asked here to coach and provide some supplies.

"I agree. Some of the young warriors are furious about it, but I think it will benefit the herd." They walked for a short distance in silence before he asked, "Do you really know so much?"

Bryan started to laugh but caught himself. The innocence in the large brown eyes told him that there was no insult hidden in the words.

"I know a lot. I am sure you know as much about your territory, about where to graze, the paths of the predators to avoid, and the lessons of the land."

Moss thought on this for a time, seeming to struggle with the terminology. "I see. Do you mean territory is meant as a possession of land?"

"Yes. Do you not consider this land yours? Others do and avoid crossing through it without consulting your elders."

"This is a lowlander error. We own nothing. The land is ours as we are the lands." It was a finite and ultimate definition, an integral meaning of life sort of statement.

"I think I agree with you. But many creatures consider an area their home, so you can also see how some who cannot migrate and wander, who stay in one place their whole life, would feel as you do about the whole?"

"Interesting. I like you, Doctor. You are brave of thought."

Before he had a chance to thank the elk, they rounded a bend, revealing dozens and dozens of tents, with elk of all shapes and sizes wandering among them. The very faint smoke of dung campfires sent small trails, adding to the mists of the morning still clinging to the dip in the high mountain valley.

Doctor Bison had never seen anything like it. He couldn't have even imagined such a gathering, not in scale or in style. The fabrics were unique; shocking even. It was more of a single type of animal he had ever seen in one place, and they flowed with a natural rhythm, all seeming to know their duty, their place.

And there must be close to five hundred elk here.

"Ah, you are impressed, with good reason." Moss chortled a free-spirited laugh.

"I am, but—"

"Three tribes are gathered here. It shocked even the young with this number of tribes folk."

"I see. That tracks better with what I know of elk herds. Still, I am impressed. Your people are vast. And so well at ease, mingling with one another."

He could tell just by looking at the small community that everyone worked and played to benefit everyone else. They wasted nothing. Everyone contributed. Not an elk was at odds with another.

"We have many customs to keep the peace, but it is a rule that everyone must give to the all. And we all desire to do so."

As they wandered down into the yurts, many small calves ran

out giggling to greet the doctor and the young warrior. He was enchanted by how careless and happy they all seemed, even the elders, the women doing their knitting, weaving.

There didn't appear to be very many male elk around other than the young warriors and the small calves, but this seemed to remind him of something he had read regarding the elk tribes and how they segregated in some ways.

The warrior led him indelibly through without pausing until they reached a smaller circle in the center.

"Here you are, doctor. This is where you will be staying." Moss backed away from the circle with the utmost respect, never turning around until he was out of sight. The doctor got the impression that he was being awarded an special honor of some kind.

Bryan idled at the edge of the circle for a bit, unsure of what he should do. He was about to seek out another elk to ask when a bent and withered little old elk lady emerged from one of the tents in the circle, moving achingly slow. She leaned on her cane, taking each step carefully, purposefully.

She came up alongside him, glancing sideways, almost as if he wasn't there.

Doctor Bison stayed very still, waiting for a cue.

"You are the doctor." The old woman stated mildly.

"I am," Bryan hesitated. The elk cow exuded a sense of authority that set him off balance.

"No."

"No?"

"Your title is only that. Simple. Meaningless. The truth of who you *are* is much more. You are a healer. You are a caretaker. You are a caregiver."

The words rang through him, a dissonant chord against his

pride, but somewhere deep inside, he felt a resonance. She was not wrong. It still made him uncomfortable.

Unsure how to reply, he offered, "I can go ahead and see to anyone who needs immediate treatment, or we can organize some group checkups, if you'd like."

"Hmm. Impatient." The old woman cocked her head to the side, raising an eyebrow.

"Or outpatient, whatever the situation calls for," Bryan blurted without thinking.

A tiny pause followed his words. Then the old cow huffed a loud and wheezing cackle, throwing her head back in laughter. Recovering, she narrowed her eyes at him. "Humor. Good. But you use it too often to avoid becoming your own patient."

Bryan choked on his own laugh. The statement was an awakening deep within.

She nodded, pointing at his flabbergasted face. "We will see to the truth in who you are. Now, we work. Come."

And with that, she abruptly led him through the circle and out into an area beyond where canopies were set up, benches and cots under the awnings. He realized at some point later in the day that he had not even asked the elder's name, or given his own, but soon overheard enough to know that everyone else called her Neinoo, which he gathered was as a much a title, and a term of endearment, as it was a name.

They saw to the ails and aches of the tribe, in no particular order of age or status. The work was steady, meaningful, and the tribe was extremely grateful to Doctor Bison. He helped carry water; he played games with the calves; he sipped tea with the elders when the sun reached its zenith in the shade of a rock formation. He even helped prepare the evening meal with the mothers and calves.

At the end of the first day, they led him to a yurt where he slept the deep sleep of exhaustion, dreaming strange dreams of endless heavens and barren mountain peaks, clouds rushing by, stars streaking behind the turn of the sky,

The coming days repeated the routine, and he came to know many across the three tribes, names, faces, tales of their journeys and the migration routes of the tribe. Through it all, Neinoo watched him, rarely offering anything but a guiding word, or comparing methods of treatment. The healers of the Stoneherd were impressively knowledgeable.

The tribe was wholesome, comforting, and lacking for nothing.

One difference in each of the following days was the meal in the evening, where he spent time among the medicine women. They directed him to sit a bit outside their close-knit group. This was always succeeded by meditation around the coals in Neinoo's large tent.

"Each passage of the sun consists of activity, sleep, and replenishment. A cycle of the sphere—light and dark. Not just those two, however. There is the dawn, and the dusk. There is the hottest part of the day, where one must seek shelter, and there is the coldest part of the dark where one needs the warmth of companionship. These things complete the circle. This is the natural order. The natural order is continuous. When we neglect a stage in our inner cycle, we stumble, we become imbalanced."

Bryan listened closely as Brush, one of the medicine cows, spoke. He ventured a question, "And what of catastrophes, storms, fires? Those upset the balance."

She smiled softly, knowingly. The question was somewhat rhetorical. "To our short-lived perception, perhaps. But that is also part of the endless cycle of the land. Fire burns, storms cleanse. What dies will be replaced and grow again. Just like when unpleasant things happen in your life. It is an upheaval, but you grow as a result."

"How do I find what is out of balance?"

"That is why we spend time looking inward, to know ourselves like we know the land. To find where the hollows are, to fill them up, to strengthen them and make ourselves whole."

"It feels very confusing."

"Nature is complex, but also simple. You learn all the working of the body. How to treat them. Why then, do you believe you cannot learn all the workings of the mind, the heart, and the spirit?"

* * *

At the end of the week, Bryan felt more rested than he had in years. He awoke every day with a spring in his step and found that his working hours were inspired. His down time gave him a surge of enjoyment, recharging him. He looked forward to each moment in the day with renewed vigor.

The tribe held a feast in his honor to see him off. Singing, dancing, and tales filled the dusk with joyous energy, and Bryan could not wait to return to Cora to share his experiences with her. He also hated the idea of leaving the tribe so soon.

As the night settled over the mountains, the young carried on in their celebrations, but the elders guided the doctor to the inner circle. There, each of the matrons sang the tale of their children, their tribe.

When the singing subsided, Neinoo took Bryan's hoof in hers and led him to a yurt he never noticed before, where each of the elder cows marked him, first with water, washing him, then with paint. Finally, a decorative gown was placed at his feet.

"You are of the Stoneherd, in your actions, and in your heart. You may come to us any time, and we would welcome you again soon, if possible."

"I am honored, Neinoo."

Neinoo took his face in her hands. "Who are you, bison?"

He looked down at the gown, around at the tent, the faces of the elk he had healed with, laughed with, cried with. "I am." Tears choked him up.

Neinoo smiled. "You are wind, a leader. You are water, a provider. You are fire, a teacher."

Bryan nodded, his heart singing.

"And you are stone, a mother. One of us."

Chapter Twelve

Medical Refugees

The Bison and the Fox

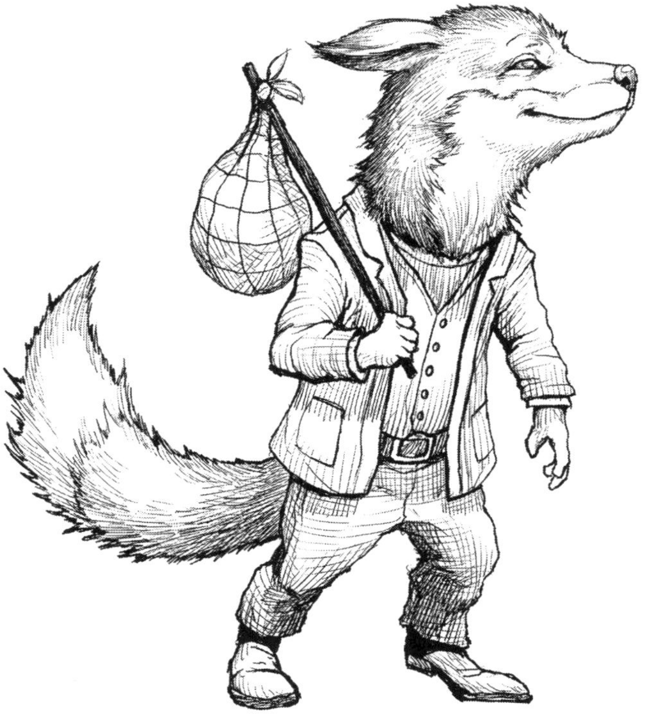

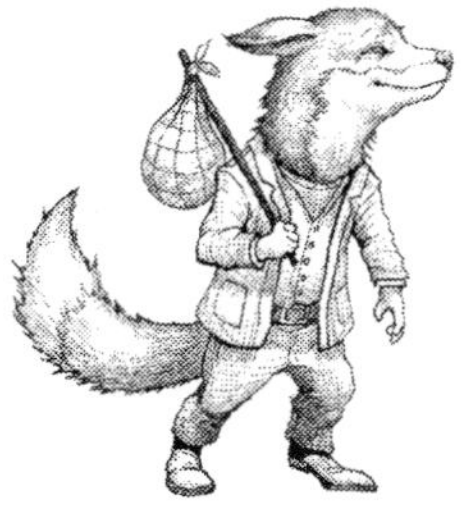

The bison had come a long and difficult way since his early days healing animals.

He previously thought that he was complete, that he had found his calling. Now, he understood the nature of healing, family, study, hard work, and physical fitness were ongoing. With this knowledge, he had found a balance to his life that he had never even imagined possible.

He felt prepared for anything life might bring.

So it was that an old animal acquaintance came to the valley, desperate for help. The fox was shunned at first, being mangy and feared to be carrying disease.

But the doctor saw the fox and recognized him and told the other animals, "Please let him enter."

After he had seen to the fox's ailments, the bison asked the fox, "Why have you come such a long-distance friend? What has happened?"

The fox broke down crying. "Everything has gone wrong. The weasel has ruined everything. All the animals you left behind are suffering and there is no one to help them."

After hearing the news, the bison grieved for his friends. He had found his own safe place, but in doing so, had left behind animals to fend for themselves.

From his place of security and healing, he realized he had the means and the obligation to do something about it. So, the bison resolved to return with his newfound abilities and right a wrong.

Once one has helped themselves become strong, they can help others.

"EXCUSE ME, DOCTOR?"

"Yes, Nurse?" Bryan looked up from the mountain of papers on his desk.

"There's a patient checking in. We're doing vitals and preliminary, but he asked for you."

The request wasn't unusual. Many repeat visitors knew their preferred doctor, and many newcomers had heard of Louis and himself over the past couple of years.

"Certainly. I'll be happy to see them."

"He says you know him." Nurse Squirrel shrugged, heading back out and down the hall.

"Hmm. Well, I do know a lot of animals," Doctor Bison chuckled to himself. "Let's see what this is all about, then."

Just over two months had passed since his self-discovery and induction into the Stoneherd tribe. Since then, he had visited every other week to spend time among the healers. Two of the times he even brought Cora along to experience the ways of his newfound folk, and to share herbal remedies between his apothecary friend and the expert traditions of the elk. Cora was just as taken and fascinated with them as he was and just as welcomed by the high mountain dwellers.

At all hours, even as he walked down the hall toward the examination room, Bryan found himself settling into a meditative state. He assessed himself frequently, his mental state, his physical state. Breathing deeply and rhythmically had become a natural part of his moment-to-moment life, and he was far less stressed, less preoccupied. The lessons of the medicine mothers were changing his anxious tendencies of overthinking and worrying into productive energy.

He had learned many things integral to his craft, as well; medicines of the land, medicines of the mind, meditation and treatments that had nothing to do with herbs or powders or food but of changing a patient's lifestyle. This behavioral and habitual adaptation of healing tied in spectacularly with the sciences of nutrition that Louis Labrador studied, as well.

Together, the teachings of the tribe melded with modern medicine, leading to spectacular discoveries and renewed ancient botanical knowledge passed down through the generations.

"Thank you for coming, Doctor. The patient is distressed." The look of discomfort on Nurse Squirrel's normally jovial face told the doctor something was truly amiss.

From the doorway, Bryan caught a look at the creature before entering. The poor, raggedy, and disheveled animal was barely recognizable as a fox. He sat on the table, fidgeting and muttering to himself, scratching at dry patches of furless skin, shaking occasionally and staring vacantly at the floor. What struck the doctor most, and was likely the source of the nurse's distress, was the look in the fox's eyes.

It was hungry. Starving. The hollow gaze reminded him with a shiver of the cougar who had chased him through the mountains.

Just a few months back, he might have mistaken it for dehydration, or the glassy look of mild fever. But he now noticed things, deeper tells in those suffering from pain and anguish, things he had felt, and things he explored in his introspection. Fear. Desperation. Longing for relief.

Still, he moved slowly, watching for reactions, on the off chance that the poor animal had contracted rabies or distemper. Despite their strides in vaccines, many rural animals did not have access to those lifesaving preventatives.

"Hi, what's your name?" Dr. Bison said softly, smiling as he took his seat. The fox flicked hesitant eyes up towards the doctor, shivering.

When his eyes fell on Dr. Bison, they lit up slightly. A flicker of life returning to the animal. "Oh, Doc Bryan. It's *so* good to see you." The comment was familiar, friendly, but also pleading.

Horror dawned on Bryan as he realized who sat before him. The fox was far from home—Bryan's old home.

"Felix?" The doctor schooled the tears of compassion that wanted to well up in his eyes. Being better in touch with his emotions made him stronger, but so too was his ability to regulate them and place them aside when necessary.

"Yessir. I heard you were practicing out this way. Had to see you."

"Of course. What brings you all the way to the mountains?"

"You," the fox's voice shook. He was emaciated, like he hadn't eaten in days traveling over a hard road. There was more, though—suffering.

"Well, I am glad you made it. It's good to see you, Felix. If you're up to it, why don't we head down to the cafeteria and get you some food. Are you thirsty, hungry?"

The question was rhetorical. He was already helping the pitiful creature to his feet, leading him out the door. His intuition told him there wasn't a dire need to check the fox for physical ailments, at least not before he was fed and rehydrated.

After getting the fox settled down at a table with a bowl of stew and some bread, and a rather large glass of water, Dr. Bison eased into the seat across from him. He smiled and nodded for Felix to eat and drink.

With that permission, the fox dove into his meal, gulping down mouthfuls of stew. As he finished his bread and most of the stew, the fox paused, looking embarrassed.

"I'm sorry, Doc. I don't mean to be so rude."

"That's alright. Just slow down a bit. Your stomach might protest so much food so soon."

Felix slowed some, chewing and closing his eyes to savor it. The cafeteria was not fine dining, but Mr. Jack Rabbit was very talented at making a lot out of a little. Yet another example of frontier living that made Doctor Bison proud.

The fox's demeanor seemed to have calmed, and he did not look so fragile, so Bryan asked, "Do you want to share with me what's happened, Felix? You've come a long way, and I might venture to assume it's not with your peddlers' wagon."

The Fox nodded slowly, a haunted shadow in his gaze.

"Doc, things have gotten really bad. You know I got around, all over, selling and trading. But I got hurt. Saw the doctor in town. They gave me some *things* to help."

The doctor nodded. He could clearly see some degenerative signs of chemical dependency. He didn't press that issue immediately, fearing that the fox might shut down or become defensive.

Felix clenched his paws, bolstering his resolve. "They started giving everyone who had the Security Plan medicine for pain. Like it was the only solution. Broken leg? Go get some powder, get some capsules. I saw it happen to lots of other folk, like it happened to me.

Ran low on funds. Couldn't afford more medicine, couldn't afford the security. So, we ran out."

A sinking feeling filled the pit of Bryan's stomach.

"There was a fella that some of us heard of. Hush, hush. Said he could get us more meds. So, I went to see him. That stuff, it felt great. Made all my woes vanish. But then . . ."

Bryan patted the air as the withered animal struggled to finish the sentence. "I understand. Did you try to see the doctor, to get advice on how to recover from the bad medicine?"

"There wasn't anyone to see, most of the time, Security or not."

"What do you mean?"

"Well, see, they had a bunch of different doctors come through there in the past couple of years. Mayor Weasel promised consistent care. Every one of them only stuck around for a short time. They'd get fed up with the system, or get run off, like what happened to you."

"What about Mister Mason? He sponsored the doctor's office. Has anyone gone to see if he could help?"

"Nobody's seen him in a while. Mayor Weasel is holed up in his mansion. And his thugs enforce the system. They police the whole town now. People who don't follow the new rules or pay up, they make examples of folks. Everyone else just goes hungry, stays sick. Nobody wants to cause a stir."

"Thank you for sharing with me, Felix. I'm so sorry. But I'll tell you what, we will get you back to your old self in no time. Let's get you a bed and Doctor Louis will give you something very mild to help you get some rest to start with."

And I will write to Nurse Rabbit and see if I can't figure out what is really going on.

Felix hugged the doctor as they stood. The bison patted his old friend on the back. He knew from experience, weaning off a drug would be difficult, but could be done.

* * *

Mister Pigeon arrived with the post late in the day. The letter was crinkled, but the writing on the front was familiar. Bryan opened the envelope slowly, anxious about what might be in the nurse's response. It had been over a month since he sent his message. He wandered back into his office, unfolding the parchment.

My dearest Doctor Bison,

I cannot tell you how good it is to hear from you and know that you are well. All of us miss you greatly. The kids all send their hellos and best wishes. Jenine insisted I share that she will be going to medical school as soon as she finishes her home studies. I wonder where that girl got her adventurous spirit.

I realize neither of us has kept up with our correspondence as well as we should have over the years, but I am so glad to hear things are still progressing well at the hospital. Someday, I swear I must make the trip to see this wonderful place you have found.

That, of course, must wait for more favorable "weather." Things at home are tough.

I carried on as long as I could, but I was, and am, very limited in my capacities. I kept the practice open even though we went through four doctors over the past two years. They are saying that no one else will come.

We are scared, Bryan. So many folks are going to court and getting thrown in jail. I was lucky enough to get off with a warning all those years back. My luck was bound to run out eventually.

Last week, Mister Ferrett suspended me, pending an investigation. I won't go too far into detail, but essentially, they made a new law outlawing some of the medicine we use. And now they are trying to say that every time we used it in the past counts as an infraction.

There is talk of jailing anyone who took it. It's madness.

We need help. Mister Mason, and many others, are in a lot of pain and suffering every day. There is no one to help them now that I cannot practice.

I am sorry to vent all of this to you, and I wish there was better news. It would mean the world to us to hear from you again. If there is anything you know of that we can do for any of the animals here, please let me know.

Sincerely,

Rebecca Rabbit

Bryan sagged in his chair, absorbing the words like physical blows. How could things have gotten so bad? Hopelessness threatened to rise up and swallow him. He was unable to offer his old friends anything from the new hospital.

His time in the mountains had been some of the best times of his life. The hospital was thriving. He was happy. In a better state of mind, body, and spirit than he had ever been. He was comfortable.

And there were creatures he could help. Creatures he *would* help.

Chapter Thirteen

The Hole and the Way Out

The Bison and the Moose

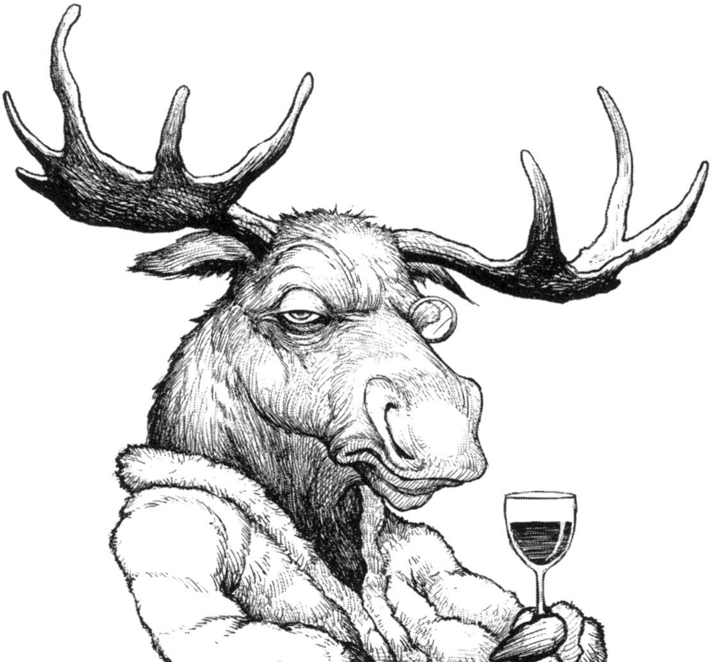

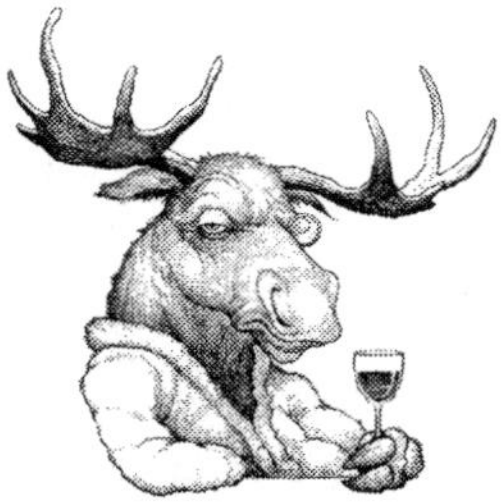

The moose suffered great pain in the years since the bison saw him last. The medicines that he received to stop the pain had become a burden. When those medicines were no longer available, the moose turned to alternative means—anything he could get to ease his pain.

Without the moose's provision to the community, things began to fall apart.

Aggressive animals stepped in to control the other animals and establish order. The bison returned to find creatures held hostage in their homes.

"Please," begged the moose, "you must help them. I will do everything I can to assist you if you will help me ease my pain."

The bison agreed, having returned to do just that. So, he helped any creature he could in secret, traveling among the animals in the darkness of night.

Before long, the animals in charge got wind of what the bison was doing. They set a trap and captured him. The weasel sneered at the bison, saying, "The moose told me you returned, trying to play the hero."

The bison became angry at the betrayal, but as he thought about it, he could not blame the moose who was suffering like the rest of the animals. In such a dire situation, animals would fight for their lives.

As a healer, however, the bison's resolve was to help those in need and sacrifice to do so.

So, the bison went with the predators to bide his time and form a plan to save the community.

Taking a stand requires taking risks.

BRYAN TIED OFF THE SPLINT, trying to be as gentle as possible. Unfortunately, it required a fair amount of force to keep the bones in place, and Buck cried out through gritted teeth.

"You're doing great, Buck. Almost there."

A final tug on the ties clenched the two boards in place, and the family, as well as Doctor Bison, sighed collectively. Deadre Deer rubbed her husband's back, tears in her eyes. She nodded with a quivering lip at the doctor.

"Thank you so much, Bryan. He's been in so much pain, and there hasn't been a thing we could do."

"You are very welcome, Deadre. I'm just sorry I wasn't around to set it before it partially healed."

Buck chuckled nervously, clearly reliving the rebreaking of his bone. His eyes were still a bit glassy from shock. "S'alright, Doc. Better than windin' up lame."

Bryan dug through his pack, drawing out a small pouch of capsules. "Take two of these per day. The injection I gave you should take care of any infection, but I want to be sure."

He packed up the rest of his tools, frowning at his dwindling supplies. Moving toward the door, Deadre cleared the way for him, but placed her cloven hoof on his arm, stopping him from leaving.

"Doctor, you are welcome to stay the night. It's very dark out there."

"I appreciate the offer, Mrs. Deer, but it's best if I don't stay in one place too long, and certainly not where I just assisted someone who shouldn't have access to care." he winked at her conspiratorially.

"We won't whisper a word."

"I know. But eventually someone is going to notice Buck back at work."

The cool evening was showing all the signs of fall's approach, but Bryan welcomed the chill after laboring over the broken leg for several hours. He constantly marveled at how easy hiking was at this lower altitude after so long in the mountains.

To keep his bearings, he kept the river on his right side, a sure means of avoiding getting close to town and the unpleasant welcome he might receive there from Mayor Weasel's enforcers. After about an hour, he spotted the dim candle in the loft of the barn. It was a marker, one that was spreading through the population, an offer of a safe place to spend the night.

Nurse Rabbit and several of the other bolder animals had developed the system, keeping her and her family safe as she continued to care for those in need. Now, the same system was gaining traction as word of the Doctor's return spread quietly throughout the countryside.

Every creature in the territory lived in a state of hyperawareness and tension. Neighbors were careful of who they said what to, fearing who might turn them in to the authorities and risk being fined, taking what little money they had left.

Work was sparse, controlled. Only the absolute necessities persisted in town.

Bryan discovered the main reason why his second day back.

He had been looking for alternate locations, potential hidden spots where he might hole up, or even set up a clinic of sorts to serve anyone who could make it to him. When he arrived at the old, abandoned copper mine, he stumbled over a mass grave. A fever, bordering on a plague, had burned through the town some months ago, likely in the spring. Later, he found out that the only response the mayor could propose was to shut down most businesses, unless it was essential for survival.

The road-worn bison slipped silently through the cracked barn door and was pleasantly surprised to find fresh straw in a stall at the back to lie on. Compared to the past several days of lying on cold, hard ground, the mound of soft, warm straw felt luxurious by comparison.

As his eyelids drooped from exhaustion, he plotted out the coming day, who he might seek out for information, who might need treatment, and where he would spend the coming night.

This is Old Collie's barn so I could try . . . sleep took him in mid thought.

* * *

"She practically handed out the prescriptions like candies at the fair." Rebecca shook her head, ears flopping before they drew right back against her head in anger. "But there was just too much backlog. Critters were waiting weeks to see her with ills that got worse from neglect."

"And then they suspended her for alleged malpractice, as if those cases that got dropped in her lap were her fault," Bentley, her husband, finished. "The so-called investigation is ongoing. Poor thing is still locked up in the pen, far as we know."

"So, Doctor Crane effectively got all of those folks hooked on pain powders. Then they were just left to drown once the doses ran out?" Bryan's shoulders sagged.

Felix Fox had not been exaggerating. If anything, it was far worse than he had relayed because a few months had passed since that encounter.

"Well, except for those that took their news to that ol' muskrat. He passes through every few weeks. Deals out poison. Got half the town hooked on the tar," Bentley spat.

The three refugees sat in a small grove of trees, sharing what news they had gathered. Using the techniques Bryan learned from the elk, they were enjoying a warm meal for a change, and the blessed heat from the nearly smokeless dung fire.

"With my supply of alternative medicines running out, it may put us in a position to contact such a creature." Doctor Bison shrugged as Rebecca scowled. "You know as well as I do that in our paws and hoofs, some of those dangerous drugs would serve just fine for what we need. It's folks self-medicating that's the real threat."

"There has to be a way to get safe and reliable supplies."

"I am all ears, Rebecca."

"Maybe we go to Mason Moose? Quietly. He's one of those I hear tell that's been in a bad way. Muskrat's been sighted stopping by his mansion more than once. It's the only sign that the mogul is still kicking." Bentley spread his paws at a loss.

"That might be our best bet. I have some of the cannabis oil that the Opossums gave me. It will help him deal with the withdrawals. Perhaps if I can palliate his issues, we can secure some funds, maybe get in contact with some of Mason's contacts in the city or find a private trader."

"It's so risky, Bryan."

"I know. But that's what I came back to do. Go be with the kids, Bent, Becca. They need you, now."

Rebecca put on a brave face, squaring her shoulders. "That's not the model I want to set for them. No, I can still help."

Bentley rested a paw on his wife's shoulder. "He might be right, darlin'. The youngins can't stay at the Mole's forever."

A silent agreement settled over the gathering. They spent the rest of the time drinking tea, reliving the old days and happier memories. The very things that made what they had set out to do worth doing.

When the bison left, they did not say goodbye.

* * *

The manor house was dark, unguarded.

It set off a warning in the Doctor's mind, raising the fur on the back of his neck. Even on the outskirts of town, Bryan felt the palpable presence of oppression, worry, and fear. But he needed to see Mason, to find out if he could offer them supplies or not. He had questions of his own. Why had the magnate abandoned the town to Weasel and his goons? At least for the sake of his financial interests.

His hoofs faltered slightly as he stepped onto the porch. This town needed him. He would not back down or run away again.

The bison bolstered his resolve, mastering his misgivings. Time in the mountains exposed him to some of the worst situations of his life, and also the best. He treated fatal wounds, saved friends' lives, and performed surgeries he had to make up on the spot, without a second to doubt his skills or instincts.

Knocking on the door twice, he waited.

After a few minutes, he was about to knock again, when the door creaked open, a sullen, small creature back lit by a single candle, stood in the foyer. Moose's assistant, Mister Ferrett, looked haggard, all rubs and sagging fur. His only reaction was a slight widening of the eyes, but whether it was shock at seeing the bison, or a warning, Bryan couldn't tell.

"C-come in."

Cobwebs and dust lined the floor and surfaces of the once pristine and opulent home. Sheets covered the paintings, and every door they passed was shut, as if to block out the world. It reminded Bryan of the mausoleums he had seen down near the coast during his training residency. The place was stale, lifeless.

But Mason had hosted guests recently. Paw prints lined the walkway to the dining hall, along the same path that Mister Ferrett now led the doctor.

"It really is good to see you, Bryan." A hollow, weak voice echoed from the back of the dim room, from the other end of the long table. "I hoped you would come."

"Mason?"

From the shadows, the once enormous animal shuffled, wrapped in a blanket. Even through the gaps in his wrap, Bryan could tell the moose was wasted, withered. His antlers had not grown back properly after the past winter, hinting at malnutrition, or chronic illness.

"Do not look at me like that, like I am to be pitied."

"I don't pity you, Mason. But I brought you something that might help."

"Help? Ha. I do not need anyone's help."

"Are you sure?"

There was an uncomfortable pause, and a flicker flashed across Mason's features. Regret. Or maybe bitterness.

"I am sorry, my old friend," Mister Moose muttered in a dry monotone. "But I will be getting the best care that money can buy. Soon."

"And who promised you that, Mason?"

"I did." Weasel stepped from another entryway, a couple of large coyotes at his back. "In exchange for turning in the rogue ex-doctor who has been practicing illegal medicine all over my territory."

Chapter Fourteen

Do No Harm

The Bison and the Herd

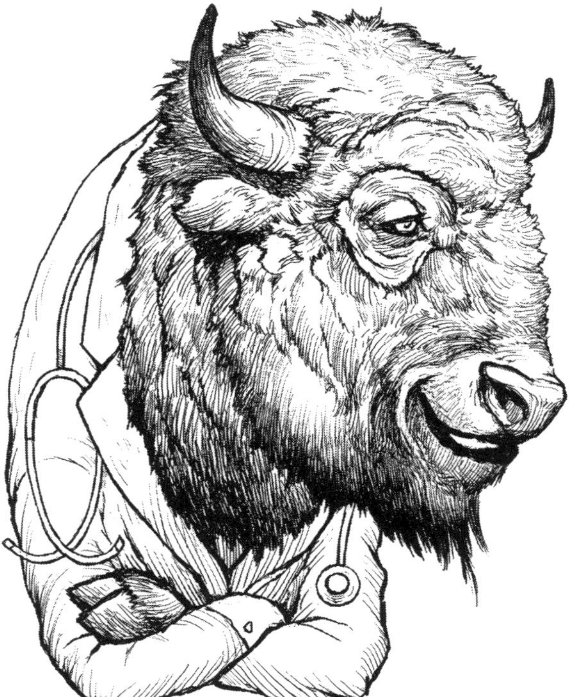

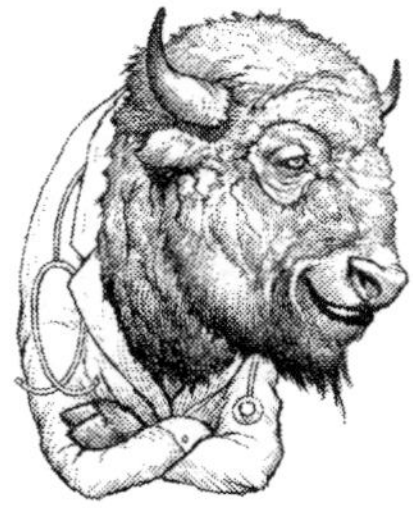

The bison found himself tied to a post on the outskirts of the community.

He was hungry and alone, but he had been through many difficult things, some much worse.

Eventually, he knew the cruel animals in charge would decide his fate, what they would do with him, or to him. He would be cast out or killed. This was the risk he took by coming back.

So it was that late one night he awoke to violent sounds and a great noise coming from beyond the hill. He waited for hours in fear for someone to come to take him or bring him some news.

Early in the morning, creatures came, many of them bloodied and bruised. But instead of harming him, they set him free and bowed to him.

"We are sorry that we cast you out, bison. We regret we didn't stand up with you," said the crow.

And the otter said, "Those animals scared us into accepting prison chains, and we took out our fears on you."

The bison told them, "I do not hold any grudges against you for trying to survive."

So, the animals asked, "Will you help us? There are many injured. We have overthrown the weasel and the predators, and we could use the help of one who knows how to provide and to heal."

Looking out over the dirty and matted faces, seeing the hope in their eyes, the bison smiled and said, "Of course, my friends. That is what healers do."

Those who would heal must not simply avoid hurting, but actively do good.

VERY LITTLE NEWS REACHED BRYAN as he sat huddled against the back wall of an old, bar-windowed wagon. The contraption hadn't been used in years, but Mayor Weasel wanted to keep him isolated, preventing as much interaction as possible with the other prisoners in the overcrowded cells at the courthouse.

The makeshift cell was cold and damp, but Bryan was well furred, so they let him keep his coat. He could have done without the shackles, and felt they were absurd because he was a powerful animal.

A short walk away, Alan Aardvark stood guard at a small campfire. The quiet former constable was an old acquaintance, his family having visited Dr. Bison's old practice in the years prior. Alan clearly took issue with the current situation, particularly in the treatment of his prisoner's condition. But he didn't dare speak out against the thugs in Weasel's employ for fear of bodily harm and the security of his family.

Good folks do what they must. Especially parents. And even more so when it seemed like the only way to feed your family properly was to work for the mayor.

Doctor Bison thought he could relate in some ways. All the animals he ever treated felt like his own children. He knew it was not entirely comparable, but in his heart, his desire to adopt anyone in pain burned brighter than ever.

A soft, sad voice inside longed for the mountain hospital as he sat curled up against the cold. Things were simpler. Those country folk were far more concerned with getting by, and helping their neighbors get by. Patients were allowed to exchange food or goods for medical care if they didn't have the money to pay.

That's all he really hoped to bring with him back to his old life.

Now, it seemed he might never get the chance to show these townsfolk a better way. Rumor had it that his trial would be fast tracked, that they would make him an example.

Regardless, he thought. I took a stand. I made a difference to a few who needed me. Maybe it will spark change.

Alan rattled the chains on the cage, alerting Bryan of his presence. He dozed off at some point and now sat up to receive the paltry plate of boiled oats shoved through the gap in the door. It was early morning, dawn a faint blue streak on the horizon.

"Thank you, Alan." The stern aardvark looked more disheveled than usual. "Any news?"

Alan simply shook his head but hesitated as he turned away. "Trouble's brewing. Don't know exactly what, but everyone is on high alert. Mayor's in a panic. I had to share my food with you this morning. They didn't come to relieve me, just sent a youngin' to tell me to stay put."

Bryan felt like there was more but did not want to press. Alan was his only tentative ally in this, and his only way out if it came down to escaping with his life.

The day crawled by, staying chilly, even more so for the strange stillness that settled over the plains. There was a tension quivering in the air, causing the crickets to go silent. Not even a breeze shifted the leaves on the nearby bushes.

And so, the bison waited, the sinking nervousness and worry seeping into his skin, curdling his stomach. Something was very wrong. Overcome with stress, he fell into a restless sleep.

At sundown, he was startled awake by a massive crash and a great rising of voices coming from over the hill. He stood up and peered through the bars, trying to see any movement in the deepening dusk when Alan came running, covered in dust and soot. The normally reserved creature was frantic, panicked. Tears streamed down his face, whether from emotion or the smell of acrid smoke that bit into Bryan's nostrils. Suddenly, he was afraid.

"Alan, what's going on?"

But the constable was a mess, tearing up his campsite, looking for something, muttering to himself. Bryan caught bits of it here and there.

"A revolt! Good folk tearing up the town. Should be doin' all we can do to keep them from hurting each other."

"Alan, snap out of it," Bryan shouted as loud as he could.

The aardvark stopped short, looking up from his daze. Then he deliberately walked to the wagon and unlocked it, opening the door.

Bryan stared at him, uncertain. "Don't put yourself or your family at risk for me, Alan. I'll be fine."

"No. Ain't right, any of it. They set up the gallows. They were going to drag you out, kill you. That's when the whole town went crazy. They stormed the mayor's mansion."

Bryan's jaw dropped. It was an honest to goodness revolution. Alan helped him as he crawled from the wagon, his legs stiff from days of sitting shackled. Together, they made slow progress back to the small camp, where they shared what was left of the water in the canteen, unsure of what to do next.

"I should get to town. See if anyone needs medical attention."

"I can't let you go. If the mayor comes back with reinforcements . . ." The poor fellow shook his head, unable to make a decision.

"Wait. The mayor is gone?"

"Yup. Escaped out the back door with a hired team pulling his buggy. Has to be heading to the next town for backup. I just know it."

"Somehow, I doubt that. But Alan, you should go check on your family. I will stay here, I promise."

Alan raised his eyes to meet the doctor's gaze, as if asking for permission. Bryan smiled encouragingly.

"Get your kids and your wife and go find Nurse Rabbit if you can, or the Otters. They can get you somewhere secure until this is over."

But when would it be over? How would it turn out? From the noise reaching them from this distance, it sounded like an all-out battle taking place in the middle of town. Alan didn't give it another thought before he was running off, back toward town.

Sitting alone, wrapped in a camp blanket, Bryan felt the weight of the events settle over him. At that moment, he was not a doctor. He was not a leader. He was not anyone's hope. He was just an animal, scared, waiting for an ending, some conclusion to a catastrophe he didn't start and had no control over.

But a warm feeling washed over him, countering the fear. He thought of Cora wearing a yellow dress and a matching hat. She wanted to come with him on this trip. He almost wished she could have, but he was glad she didn't. He wanted her to be safe.

What would you say right now, my dearest friend? he thought. *You'd say, "Heaven forbid that the great and wise doctor is not the one leading the revolution. Feel sorry, but stop feeling sorry for yourself. This is who you are."*

"You're right, Cora. And Lham would tell me that these chains are only on my body and shouldn't hold my mind and heart. And Louis would tell me I am missing out on a perfectly good opportunity to finally get some good sleep by a warm fire." Bryan stoked the embers back to life, chuckling in the darkness. Soon, he was fast asleep.

* * *

Dawn spread her thin fingers of mist across the rolling grass of the plains, bringing with it a steady wind to drive away the smoke. Nothing moved in the town as Bryan stood looking down the low hill that sloped to the start of the main street.

Finally awake, he felt a pressing need to get up and move. After digging through Alan's things, he found a hammer that he used to break the pin on his ankle shackles. Then he shuffled his way back to town.

The town was in shambles.

Many buildings lay in ruin, windows broken, doors kicked in. Some had burned down completely through the night. Most notable were the courthouse and the mayor's mansion. A rising panic rippled through him as he made his way along the road.

What if they didn't get the animals in the cells out before it all collapsed on them?

Steady, Doctor. Don't lose it, now.

He took a deep breath and took control of his wild thoughts, forcing them to mimic the calm of the operating room. Taking another deep breath, he suddenly smelled food.

A laugh of disbelief huffed from his hefty chest as he spotted something else ahead, waving in the breeze outside of the town meeting hall. Hung for anyone to see from all over town, a white banner with a red cross painted crudely on either side flapped gently from side to side.

It was a wartime call to those who needed help, who needed care and a place to rest.

The doors to the hall were wide open, one of them barely hanging from the shattered hinges. As he stepped into the open doorway, he saw the extent of the horrors that had befallen his little town. Dozens of citizens were laying on makeshift cots, or simply blankets laid out on the floor. Others sat on benches, in chairs, or leaned against the walls. Everywhere he looked, there were injuries. Burns, scrapes, broken bones, some far worse, and still others from blunt force traumas, likely from the mayor's guards, none of whom seemed to be present any longer.

"Doc?" a familiar voice called out, as a young rabbit trotted down the aisle. "Doc, is that you?"

"Jenine?" Bryan gaped. She was the spitting image of her mother, and she had grown a foot since the last time he'd seen her.

"Oh, thank goodness. There isn't . . . I mean, I know a lot of basics that Momma showed me, but . . ."

"Is Rebecca alright? Your father, your brothers?" Panic threatened to rise again.

"They are fine, but Momma fainted from exhaustion. Poppa's about as bad. They worked throughout the night after the fighting died down."

By this time, other animals started stirring and murmuring at the doctor's presence. Many looked ashamed, some hopeful, others wary. *Did they think he caused all of this?*

Bryan looked from one animal to the next, lost in recollections, memories, lost in the horrors he saw before him, and the hurt that this town had inflicted on him. Tears filled his eyes, choked him up. He was still angry, all things said and done. Sad. Frustrated. Confused.

Jenine gripped his hoof, pulling him out of his mental haze. He looked down, noting the open worry plain in her matted, soot-stained face. So too, there was relief, and true caring in those eyes. "I'm just so glad you're alive, Uncle Bryan. We all are."

And then, the sadness was gone—and the anger with it.

Only one thought remained in the Doctor's mind—the words of the elk mothers. Leader. Provider. Teacher. Mother.

"Let's set up a new station over here in the entry. I'll get you a list of everything I need. You're going to make a fine nurse, Jenine."

The rabbit's face lit up, as well as did those who overheard the announcement. Someone shouted a cheer farther back in the room. Soon, animals were helping the more injured to line up and organize.

By noon, with the help of the Mice, the Otters, the Moles, and the Goose families, they had a cook tent set up, preparing rations for the whole town. By sundown, all available bedding, the rooms still usable, and the structures still sound enough to enter, were prepared for everyone to find a place to sleep.

One by one, every member of the community, injured or hale, came to the Doctor to thank him, to offer him water, food, or anything they might do for him. And more often than not, they apologized.

Doctor Bison shook each of their hands and reassured them.

Late on the second day, a silence fell over the hall as a hunched figure entered. Mister Mason entered cautiously, wary of the surrounding animals. None of them laid a paw on the moose, but many animals glared and sneered at one of the culprits of the town's downfall.

The decrepit tycoon stopped in front of the Doctor, pausing in his examination of a sprained paw. Bryan simply raised his eyebrows expectantly, noting as he did that while Mason still looked terrible, he had that old spark and fire in his eyes again. He was kicking his addiction.

"I have come to turn myself in, to fall on your mercy, Doctor. You, who I did the most wrong to, who I betrayed, I won't ask for forgiveness."

"Well, that's good, because I don't have time to give it." He chuckled, gesturing at the line of sick and injured still needing his attention. "Besides, this town has seen enough adversity. What we need now is to come together and heal. Pitch in. Get to work. Earn their trust back."

"Even after the way we treated you?" Mason exclaimed. "You'd have every right to leave all of us to our fates. Let us suffer for our crimes."

"My oath is to do no harm. But we must also choose to do *good.* We must do *more.*"

* * *

Bryan woke early, like he did most days, and headed to the new medical facilities to see what the day held. New animals began to filter into town again. Trade routes were opening back up, and farming and daily routines resumed.

This day was like every other day, and there was already a short line outside the small building when he arrived. This day was special, just like every other day. The town was on the mend after endless turmoil.

As he entered, Cora greeted him with a list of patients and their concerns. "Shall we?" she asked, smiling.

And so, the doctor entered the examination room, greeting a newcomer to the town, a beaver wearing a thick pair of spectacles. The critter blinked up at the looming bison, a bit shocked.

"Good morning. Thomas, is it? I'm Bryan, I'll be your doctor."

The beaver nodded cordially, adjusting his spectacles. "Nice to meet you, Bryan. So, what kind of doctor are you if you don't mind me asking?"

"A really good one."

EPILOGUE

My life has been a kind of Native American pathfinding adventure on Mother Earth.

"Listen to the wind, it talks. Listen to the silence, it speaks. Listen to your heart, it knows."

I am attracted to everyone, as the possibility exists that I have a contribution for them. During my exploration of how we might get related, I serve their spirit and soul by honoring who they are deep inside. I was into healing before I became a physician. That is one of the prime sources of my enlivenment. It is in my DNA to relieve those I encounter from their pain.

My soulmate, Susan Franzheim, became my coach when it was darkest before the dawning of the possibility of living my best life. She related to my travails with the "powers-that-be." She advised, "No one on Earth can take away from you, your mission to serve and heal. When you were trapped and forced to relinquish your clinic, you assisted the Dalai Lama in opening his clinic in Zanskar, India. In Calcutta, India, you worked alongside Mother Teresa. You treated Pain Refugees in Greece."

Seeking anyone who may be open to our being midwives for birthing possibilities in their lives, Susan and I were blessed to have a decade of Landmark Education's transformational courses which source our work.

Persian poet, philosopher, and lover of humanity, Rumi, wrote: "Yesterday I was clever, so I wanted to change the world. Today I am wise, so I am changing myself."

Rumi's sentiment informs my life.

ABOUT THE AUTHOR

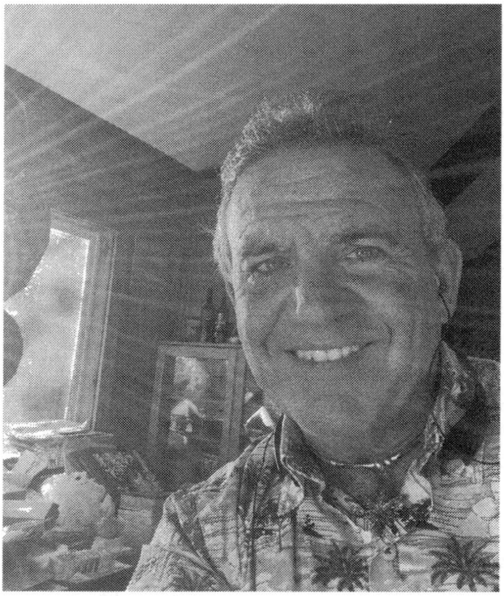

MARK IBSEN, MD has been practicing medicine for over forty years. Born in Grand Rapids, MI and raised in Geneva, IL, he was the youngest of four siblings. He dreamed of being a professional football player but stopped growing in the seventh grade. His second choice was to be a doctor.

His attended Williams College for his undergraduate work, followed by medical school at Washington University in St. Louis, Missouri. His residency in family medicine took place at University of Utah from 1980 to 1983. His post graduate medical and communication education includes bedside, ultrasound, tropical medicine, and ten-plus years communication training through Landmark education.

Ibsen practiced Emergency Medicine through 2012. He opened

an urgent care facility in 2010 which closed in 2015. He currently practices natural and transpersonal medicine in the realm of cannabis, ketamine, pain refugees, and end-of-life care.

Dr. Ibsen was first injured at age twelve and has lived with chronic pain since then. He has also endured degenerative disc disease, two back surgeries, ruptured Achilles tendon, carpal tunnel repair, and coronary artery bypass graft. Ibsen recognizes that his training in pain medicine in addition to his Emergency Medicine career relates directly to his personal experiences with chronic pain, giving him a unique perspective and empathy for his patients.

His other interests include wilderness exploration and refugee medicine in rural and inner-city America, as well as Nepal, India, and the Greek Islands with Syrian refugees. He has two children, Grace and Alfred.

For the interested reader regarding pain refugees, he recommends reading *Handbook to Live Well with Adhesive Arachnoiditis* by Forest Tennant, MD, MPH, DrPH.

Another valuable resource is painnewsnetwork.org.

Other books on the subject that Ibsen recommends include: *Pain in America: And How Our Government Makes It Worse!* by John P. Flannery, II

A Nation in Pain: Healing Our Biggest Health Problem by Judy Foreman

Burden of Pain: A Physician's Journey Through the Opioid Epidemic by Dr. Jay K. Joshi

The human rights issue of pain is addressed in the book *American Agony: The Opioid War Against Patients in Pain* by Helen Borel, RN, PhD.

Another valuable resource is Pain News Network (painnewsnetwork.org). It is an independent, nonprofit online news service that provides in-depth coverage about chronic pain and illness. Its mission is to raise awareness about chronic pain, and to connect and educate pain sufferers, caregivers, healthcare providers and the public about the pain experience.

For reliable information regarding chronic pain, cross-referenced and thoroughly researched, a great resource is Richard A. Lawhern, PhD and Practical Pain Management (practicalpainmanagement.com)

To become involved and have your voice heard on the issue of chronic pain, please explore:

The Doctor Patient Forum (thedoctorpatientforum.com)

The Innocence Project (innocenceproject.org)

American Council on Health and Science (acsh.org)

American Civil Liberties Union (aclu.org)

Your Senators, Representatives, and Governor

Made in the USA
Columbia, SC
21 March 2025

272b006c-7ced-4142-835c-6ee09a42fc4aR02